I0048045

# Child And Adolescent Clinical Psychopharmacology Made Simple

John D. Preton, Psyd, Abpp
John H. O'Neal, Md
Mary C.Talaga, Rph, Phd
Bret A. Moore, Psyd, Abpp

16pt

Read How You Want
LARGE PRINT BOOKS, BRAILLE & DAISY

# Copyright Page from the Original Book



Distributed in Canada by Raincoast Books


New Harbinger Publications, Inc.
5674 Shattuck Avenue
Oakland, CA 94609
www.newharbinger.com



Acquired by Jennye Garibaldi; Cover design by Amy Shoup;
Text design by Tracy Marie Carlson

Library of Congress Cataloging-in-Publication Data on file

# TABLE OF CONTENTS

"This book is remarkable in its ability to communicate essential, factual, and practical information in a concise and easily readable manner. Each chapter manages to succinctly provide the reader with information about diagnostic considerations, clinical signs and symptoms of the disorder, and the most effective and up-to-date approaches to treatment. I would recommend this book for students, professionals, individuals who live with the disorders, and their families/caregivers."

**—Joseph E. Comaty, PhD, MP,** clinical psychologist, medical psychologist (Louisiana), and coauthor of *Julien's Primer of Drug Action*

"The fourth edition of *Child and Adolescent Clinical Psychopharmacology Made Simple* presents pediatric disorders and their treatments in a highly readable and well-organized style. Not only are agents formally approved for pediatric use covered, but so are the many drugs frequently prescribed 'off-label.' Numerous tips are also included on how pediatric management both overlaps and differs from adults.

A must-read for those learning to treat children and adolescents."

—**Stephen Stahl, MD, PhD, DSc,** professor of psychiatry at the University of California, Riverside; honorary fellow of the University of Cambridge; and author of more than 500 scientific papers and sixty books on psychiatry and psychopharmacology

"This book offers a clear review of the medications used to treat the most common psychiatric conditions in children. The ample use of tables and boxes makes information such as dosing and common side effects readily accessible. Additional information about over-the-counter agents and dietary supplements—as well as patient information sheets about specific classes of medications—provides an added benefit of great practical value to both parents and early career professionals."

—**Jacobus Donders, PhD, ABPP,** chief psychologist at Mary Free Bed Rehabilitation Hospital, and coeditor of *Clinical Neuropsychology Study Guide and Board Review*

"This well-written and easy-to-read book puts at your fingertips a quick reference for those who diagnose and treat children and adolescents with psychiatric disorders. Outside of the basics, it provides the reader with a sense that the authors, outside of being experts, treat patients in their own practices and live by what they teach in their writing of this book."

**—Thomas L. Schwartz, MD,** author of *Practical Psychopharmacology,* and professor and interim chair of psychiatry at SUNY Upstate Medical University

# PRAISE FROM PREVIOUS EDITIONS

"*Child and Adolescent Psychopharmacology Made Simple* is an outstanding contribution for the non-pharmacist health professional. The chapters are clear, practical, concise, and authored by pharmacists, physicians, and behavioral health experts with current knowledge and valuable insights for health professionals working in medical, dental, and behavioral health settings."

**—William Gordon, PhD,** president of the Institute for Brain Potential

"This is a great handbook that is up to date and very clearly written. The short chapters and multiple tables make it extremely easy to use. I find it ideal when I need quick access to information on the latest psychopharmaceuticals for kids."

**—Daniel Carlat, MD,** associate clinical professor of psychiatry at Tufts University School of Medicine, and publisher of *The Carlat Psychiatry Report*

To my grandsons, Atticus and Ender: identical and so unique!

—JP

In memory of Patrick Everette Cummings.... Your spirit lives on.

—MT

To my patients, for they have been my best teachers.

—JO

To my wife Lori and her unshakable support, and daughter Kaitlyn and her perpetual inspiration.

—BAM

# Acknowledgments

Many thanks to our publisher, Dr. Matthew McKay, freelance copy editor Gretel Hakanson, and our most excellent editors, Melissa Kirk, Catharine Meyers, Karen O'Donnell Stein, and Kayla Sussell.

Thanks to our families, with deep appreciation for their patience and encouragement.

Finally, a heartfelt thanks to our patients.

May this book help our fellow mental health clinicians in our shared and ongoing struggle to reduce emotional suffering in young people.

# INTRODUCTION

# Sharing Our Concerns: For H+ealth Care Providers, Parents, and Patients

*Facts without values, fragmentary specialties with no integrating philosophy of life as a whole, data with no ethical standards for their use, techniques ... with no convictions about life's ultimate meaning ... here a panacea has turned out to be a problem.*

—Harry Emerson Fosdick
*The Living of These Days* (1956)

Many young people experience considerable emotional suffering. Oftentimes this psychological pain is associated with poverty, poor prenatal care, racial or other forms of discrimination, serious family dysfunction, traumatic life events, or any of a host of neuropsychiatric disorders. Only certain types of emotional distress are appropriate for treatment with psychiatric medications.

Psychiatric medication treatment of children and teenagers began in the 1960s. Yet only recently have large-scale medication trials been conducted. The research in child psychiatry is still considered to be limited. Clearly advances have been made, both in the safety of medications and in the development of treatment guidelines. In this book we summarize basic information regarding classes of psychological disorders for which medications are often prescribed, and we present current guidelines for the use of medications. However, we first want to state three important and overarching concerns.

The first concern is that in the current era of managed care, it is common for insufficient time or attention to be given to conducting a comprehensive history and diagnostic evaluation. Such an evaluation is essential before any recommendation can be made regarding treatment. Second, it is clear that when psychiatric medications are used to treat particular disorders, close follow-up is warranted and essential for addressing problems of treatment adherence, managing side effects, and monitoring response to treatment. Third, most children and teenagers suffering from psychological problems do not require medication treatment; instead, they may need psychosocial interventions, often involving the family as well as the individual. Even in those conditions that are judged to be largely neurobiological in nature and responsive to medication treatments, psychotherapy is *always* indicated.

In voicing these three issues, it may seem as if we are just stating the obvious; however, our concern is that with the quick-fix and get-on-with-your-life mentality in our social culture and the health care industry's focus on cost containment, the knee-jerk reaction of too many providers may be to reach for the prescription pad whenever they see psychological symptoms. While the appropriate use of psychiatric medications has helped many young people, we feel it's important for us to strongly endorse a comprehensive approach to treatment. This approach should be based on careful evaluations, close monitoring, and the use of psychotherapy, with medications prescribed only if warranted.

It is also important for clinicians, consumers, and parents alike to be aware of the risks and benefits of all treatments. Because of the enormous complexity of human psychological functioning, most problems are multidimensional and require interventions on a number of levels. And it is equally important to be humble regarding our approaches to treatment. Psychiatric drugs, as we shall see in this volume, can reduce rates of suicide, may decrease the risk of substance abuse, and in some instances may prevent certain kinds of brain damage. But medical treatments also have clear limits; there are no panaceas. No drug can mend a broken heart, fill an empty life, or teach parents how to love their children.

CHAPTER 1

# Issues in Psychopharmacological Treatment of Children and Adolescents

In this first chapter we address a number of general issues that are important to consider prior to discussing diagnosis and treatment, the specifics of which we'll cover in the chapters that follow.

## DIAGNOSING AND TREATING CHILDREN AND ADOLESCENTS

Until just recently, in child psychiatry there appeared to be an assumption that children with psychiatric disorders were quite similar, if not identical, to adults with respect to both diagnostic and pharmacological treatment issues. The recommended approach was to diagnose and treat as you would with adults, although generally starting treatment with lower doses of medications. Even though there is some degree of symptomatic overlap between adult-onset and childhood-onset disorders, there are also significant features that distinguish psychiatric syndromes as well as pharmacological treatments in children and adults. Also keep in mind that the target of psychiatric drugs (the central nervous system) is continuously undergoing maturational changes throughout childhood and adolescence. Certain neurotransmitter systems are not fully online in children, and some brain structures have not reached full development. Body characteristics (e.g., lean tissue versus body fat) change over time, which impacts how well the drug molecules are transported to where they need to be. In a sense, using psychotropic drugs with younger clients is like shooting at a moving target. Likewise, there are significant differences between adults and younger people in the way the drugs are metabolized. Even though their bodies are smaller, the kidneys and liver of children (key organs involved in processing medications) are more efficient than those of adults. Kids are not just smaller versions of adults. Their bodies handle drugs differently, and to treat a child as a "miniadult" will very likely lead to a poor outcome.

It is likely that the majority of emotional suffering experienced by youngsters is related to situational stress and responds best to nonmedical, psychological treatments (e.g., family therapy). However, it is also becoming increasingly clear that many major mental illnesses begin in childhood (for example, 25 percent of obsessive-compulsive disorder cases and up to 15 percent of bipolar disorder cases have childhood or early-adolescent onset). Not only do these disorders cause considerable suffering in young children, but they can also markedly interfere with normal social and academic developmental experiences. For example, more than one-half of children experiencing major depression continue to be symptomatic for more than 2 years. During depressive episodes, many experience significant social withdrawal and academic failure, often due to an impaired ability to concentrate. Even if they recover, many of these children find it hard to ever catch up academically or socially.

Increasing evidence also shows that some psychiatric disorders, if they go untreated, leave patients subject to progressive neurobiological impairment (the kindling model of disease progression). Toxic levels of neurotransmitters, such as glutamate, or stress hormones, such as cortisol, may damage neural tissue or interfere with normal patterns of neuromaturation (see figure 1-A). Pharmacological treatment of childhood psychiatric disorders may not only be successful in improving symptoms but also neuroprotective (in other words, medication treatment may either protect against brain damage or promote normal neuromaturation; in some instances, medications may promote the regeneration of some nerve cells, a process called *neurogenesis*).

DISORDERS WITH EVIDENCE OF PROGRESSIVE NEUROBIOLOGICAL IMPAIRMENT

- Bipolar disorder
- Attention-deficit/hyperactivity disorder (ADHD)
- Schizophrenia
- Some cases of recurrent unipolar depression
- Some cases of post-traumatic stress disorder

**Figure 1-A**

# INFORMED CONSENT AND ADDRESSING PARENTAL CONCERNS

In addition to clinical considerations, other unique challenges arise in the prescribing of psychotropic medications for children. Children cannot give true *informed consent* since parents are the ones who usually decide whether or not to allow medication treatment. This presents at least four concerns: (1) fears about drug use (or possible addiction) may lead parents to withhold treatment from some children who need it; (2) some parents may see psychiatric disorders simply as chemical imbalances, believe that pills will fix the problem, and ignore psychological factors (such as dysfunctional family dynamics) as a focus for treatment; (3) parents may use medications primarily for behavioral control despite detrimental side effects (for example, using excessive doses of stimulants to markedly reduce hyperactive behavior in children with attention-deficit/hyperactivity disorder, even though it may cause lethargy and sedation and, if doses become too high, decreased cognitive functioning); and (4) the young person is left out of the loop, perhaps not consulted about how he or she feels about medication treatment.

Most pediatric clinicians agree that children should be included in discussions about psychiatric medication treatment (especially children ages 7 and older whose cognitive development has proceeded enough that they can understand some information regarding medication treatment). Again, children cannot give consent, but they can give assent (informal expression of approval or agreement). Providing information is important in order to encourage the child to voice concerns about treatment, since many children conclude that if they need medicine, they must be very ill or "crazy." Also, these early experiences with psychiatric treatment, if perceived to be beneficial by the child, may go a long way toward instilling positive attitudes about mental health treatment (this is a critical point, since many of the more severe disorders that warrant medical treatment during childhood are the first manifestations of what may be lifelong mental illnesses). Including the child in discussions regarding medication treatment can often make him or her feel respected and thereby foster a positive relationship with the therapist or physician. At all times, when feasible, the child should be an active collaborator in the medication decision-making process as a way to increase engagement and treatment adherence.

Because parents who do not wholeheartedly endorse treatment will often sabotage it, professionals need to devote a good deal of time to addressing all of their concerns about drug treatment. Informed consent should also include the risks of not treating certain disorders.

## *Parental Fears Regarding Drug Addiction*

Many parents are understandably concerned about the use of habit-forming drugs to treat their children. It is important that clinicians talk openly with parents about these concerns (even if parents do not initiate the conversation). Among psychiatric medications, only two classes encompass potential drugs of abuse: stimulants (such as Ritalin and Adderall) and benzodiazepines (antianxiety drugs such as Xanax). However, the vast majority of children with psychiatric disorders do not abuse these medications. Although stimulants can be abused by those genetically predisposed toward substance abuse, such drugs generally do not produce euphoria in children with ADHD. In fact, many children with ADHD experience mild dysphoric effects from stimulants. Additionally, current data indicate that among those with ADHD, the use of stimulants may decrease the risk of substance abuse in comparison with drug abuse rates among nontreated ADHD subjects. Where we most often see psychostimulants abused is in high-achieving adolescents who capitalize on the energy and focus-enhancing effects of the medications to help maintain hectic academic and extracurricular schedules.

Substance abuse by children and adolescents is a common and serious concern in our society. It must also be kept in mind that untreated mental illnesses result in significant emotional suffering and contribute to a much higher likelihood of drug abuse down the line. Low self-esteem, depression, anxiety, and a sense of alienation often prompt the use of illicit drugs as a form of self-medication. Thus, any risk-benefit assessment of medication treatment and drug abuse must certainly take into consideration the risks of failure to treat the psychiatric disorder.

# MEDICATIONS AND THE MEDIA

Research studies and clinical experience certainly influence prescribing practices. However, in recent years the media have had a profound effect on public opinion and ultimately on clinical practice. Public opinion is often influenced by both drug companies' marketing efforts (and thus their profit motives) and news headlines—an example of this is the recent concern over antidepressant use in children and its possible relationship with increased suicidality, an issue discussed in more detail in chapter 2.

In the late 1980s, negative attention was focused on the drug Ritalin (methylphenidate), a widely prescribed stimulant used to treat ADHD. Andrew Brotman (1992), summarizing the work of Safer and Krager (1992), states, "The media attack was led by major national television talk show hosts and in the opinion of the authors, allowed anecdotal and unsubstantiated allegations concerning Ritalin to be aired. There were also over twenty lawsuits initiated throughout the country, most by a lawyer linked to the Church of Scientology."

In a study conducted in Baltimore, Maryland, examining the effects of this negative media and litigation blitz, Safer and Krager found that during the 2-year period just following the negative media attention, prescriptions for Ritalin had dropped by 40 percent. What were the consequences? Of those children who discontinued use of Ritalin, 36 percent experienced major academic maladjustment (such as failing grades or suspension) and another 47 percent had mild to moderate academic problems. During this time there was a 400 percent increase in the prescription of tricyclic antidepressants (TCAs), which were then being used in place of Ritalin (studies had demonstrated that TCAs were somewhat effective in treating ADHD symptoms but clearly much less effective than stimulants). Further, TCAs are considerably more toxic, have much higher rates of side effects, and have been associated with sudden cardiac-related deaths in six children. Clearly, parents had heard the negative reports about Ritalin in the media and approached their pediatricians with concerns about the drug. As a result, many children were taken off the stimulant and put on a class of drugs that was less effective and considerably more dangerous.

Media attention is important in that it can alert consumers and professionals (including the Food and Drug Administration, or FDA) to possible problems with certain medications. When this leads to more thorough investigations, sometimes drugs are found to be problematic or unsafe. However, it can also lead to unwarranted fears and ultimately to clinical decisions that may not be in the best interest of our clients. The point is that media-driven concerns raised by our clients and their parents can be significant, and we as clinicians must be aware of and sensitive to such concerns.

# DRUG RESEARCH AND OUT COME STUDIES

As important as efficacy studies are, there is a relative paucity of good studies in child psychopharmacology (with the notable exception of the numerous well-controlled studies of the treatment of ADHD with stimulants). In the past, pharmaceutical companies did not conduct tests of psychiatric drugs on children. However, in 1997 the Food and Drug Administration mandated that safety studies be carried out for new psychiatric drugs with child subjects. Moreover, in 2002, Congress passed the Best Pharmaceuticals for Children Act (BPCA) and in 2003, the Pediatric Research Equity Act. The BCPA includes a provision that offers financial incentives (in the form of extensions of patents; even a 6-month patent extension can lead to hundreds of millions of dollars in profit for a pharmaceutical company) for conducting efficacy studies with children. Thus, in very recent times, better-controlled studies have been initiated, although many of these are not yet published and some suffer from significant methodological flaws. It is hoped that in the next few years, the number of well-done studies will increase significantly.

Another concern is that many studies do not include severely ill children (the reason being that it is not considered ethical to expose severely disturbed children to placebos over a period of months). Thus, in some child psychiatry studies involving random assignment and the use of placebos, groups of subjects often include only mild to moderately severe cases. Information about treatment outcomes for severely ill kids is often limited to that which comes from clinical experience and case studies. It is important to keep these research limitations in mind when evaluating the outcomes of medication studies.

A third area of concern, both for clinicians and for parents, is the effect of very long-term use of psychiatric medications in children. Short-term side effects are well documented and will be discussed in detail in subsequent chapters. However, there is relatively little hard data that indicate the risks associated with long-term treatments. Yet, for many of the disorders discussed in this book, including bipolar disorder, ADHD, and psychotic disorders, long-term medication treatment is strongly recommended. It is our belief that when this topic arises in discussions with patients and their parents, the clinician's only appropriate response is to be completely candid about the lack of knowledge regarding long-term drug exposure, but to also be clear about the risks of not treating certain disorders. Deciding whether to use medication is always a matter of evaluating risk versus benefit, and parents need to be offered as much information as possible so they can make informed choices. Related, it is important to remember that the parent or guardian is the one who makes the decision about whether or not the child takes a medication, not the clinician. The role of the prescribing clinician is as a consultant to the parent.

# MEDICATION METABOLISM IN YOUNG CLIENTS

The normal rate of hepatic (liver) metabolism is high in children until the time of puberty. The result is that most medications are aggressively metabolized in the liver and rapidly excreted. Because what ultimately matters is how much of the drug enters the bloodstream, treatment of prepubertal children may require doses that approach or equal those for adults. (The use of seemingly high doses for young children may seem counterintuitive to many parents, and thus it will be helpful for clinicians to explain the role of increased rates of drug metabolism.) If too low of a dose is provided, the young child will experience suboptimal treatment with the potential of progressive worsening of the psychiatric condition.

During the 2 to 4 months surrounding the entry into puberty, the rate of hepatic metabolism significantly slows. For this reason, youngsters who have been on a maintenance dose of psychiatric medication and tolerating it well may begin to show increasing side effects when this change in metabolic rate occurs and more of the drug begins to escape the liver and enter circulation. Dosage adjustments may then be required, to minimize side effects. In extreme cases, if the dose is too high relative to the decreased rate of metabolism, the child may develop toxic levels of the medication in the blood leading to serious physical and neurological consequences.

## APPROVED DRUGS AND OFF-LABEL USE

Currently very few psychiatric drugs are approved by the FDA for use in treating children and young adolescents. Yet these few drugs are also in widespread use in child psychiatry. It is very common practice in the field, and in general medicine, to prescribe drugs *off label,* meaning other than as approved by the FDA. For example, the antipsychotic medication Haldol (haloperidol) is FDA approved for the treatment of schizophrenia but not bipolar disorder. However, Haldol has been used for a number of years to treat cases of mania. Another example is the use of Prozac (fluoxetine), which is approved to treat obsessive-compulsive disorder in children, but is not approved for the treatment of social anxiety disorder (social phobia). It is commonly used by clinicians for treatment of the latter in youngsters.

Since clinical and scientific research supports the use of these drugs in treating non-FDA-approved disorders, their use is considered to be in keeping with medical standards of practice, and thus neither illegal nor unethical. Likewise, many drugs approved for use in adults (but not in children) are used to treat child psychiatric patients. For example, only fluoxetine has been approved by the FDA for the treatment of major depression in children, yet many other antidepressants are used to treat childhood-onset depression.

Some drug classes, most notably antidepressants, have been found effective in treating a host of disorders other than depression, such as panic disorder, obsessive-compulsive disorder, and generalized anxiety disorders. We will discuss the use of antidepressants in more detail in chapter 2, and in later chapters we will address how such drugs play a role in the treatment of other disorders.

# ATTITUDES AND REALITIES REGARDING PSYCHOPHARMACOLOGY WITH CHILDREN AND ADOLESCENTS

Despite the fact that some of the disorders discussed in the following chapters are deemed to be largely the result of a primary neurobiological cause and require drug treatment, we categorically state, as we did in the introduction, that no child should ever be treated with psychiatric medications without concurrent psychotherapy. It is common for pediatricians to diagnose psychiatric disorders and prescribe psychotropic medications, and in very rare cases pediatricians have both appropriate training for diagnosing and treating psychiatric disorders and enough time to conduct a comprehensive evaluation. Yet the reality is that most primary care doctors are overwhelmed with patients and have grossly inadequate amounts of time to devote to taking careful histories, conducting thorough diagnostic evaluations, and providing timely, appropriate follow-up. We strongly believe that children with serious mental illnesses should be evaluated and treated by mental health specialists.

We also believe that the decision to begin a child on a psychotropic medication is not one that should be made lightly. Psychiatric medications come with risks. And as noted earlier, little information is known about the effects of these powerful medications over the long term. Therefore, we believe clinicians and parents should carefully consider whether or not medication is necessary. This may seem like an easy and straightforward question, but it's not. Understanding the impact on functioning in key areas (school, family, interpersonal) is critical.

It's important to consider whether the child can function well enough with non-pharmacological interventions or if the medication is needed to ensure a basic level of functioning is achieved. This is most relevant for those children who are on the verge of failing or being expelled from school or for those whose behavior is bringing them into contact with law enforcement. It is certainly critical for children who are battling severe depression to the point that harm to self could occur.

We believe that nonpharmacological approaches should be considered first unless there are safety concerns. And in all cases, psychosocial interventions should be an integral part of any treatment plan when a child is prescribed medication. The reality is that financial and time constraints, pressure from parents, teachers, and school administrators, and the desire of the clinician and parents to help the child as quickly as possible lead to medication as a first-line approach to care. This is not always in the best interest of the child.

# THE USE OF DSM-5 DIAGNOSTIC CRITERIA

We have incorporated criteria from *DSM-5* (*Diagnostic and Statistical Manual of Mental Disorders, Fifth Edition,* 2013); however, in many instances, we have described diagnostic criteria more briefly than can be found in *DSM-5.* This book is written both for professionals and for a lay audience (parents), and thus, we have listed criteria using language that is familiar to both types of readers. *DSM-5* contains a much more detailed description of diagnostic signs and symptoms.

# WHERE WE GO FROM HERE

In the chapters that follow, we will discuss specific classes of psychiatric disorders. The initial focus of each chapter will be on important issues regarding diagnosis, highlighting new developments in the diagnosis of childhood disorders. This will be followed by an overview of medications that are commonly used to treat particular disorders, and then specific treatment guidelines. Please note that the appendix of this book includes general information sheets regarding six common classes of psychotropic drugs that may be given to patients or used by caregivers. We believe that it is very important for consumers to become knowledgeable about treatment options and the risks and benefits of medications. Please feel free to make copies of these sheets and use them as handouts in your practice. You can also find downloadable versions of the handouts online at http://www.newharbinger.com/45120. (See the very back of this book for more information.)

# CHAPTER 2

# Depression

Accurate prevalence rates for adjustment disorders with depressed mood in children are not available, although the rates are likely to be high. However, epidemiologic studies have established that yearly prevalence rates of major depression are significant (2 percent for children and 10 percent for teenagers). Of great concern is the fact that serious depressive episodes in children and young adolescents are also likely to herald the onset of either severe and highly recurrent unipolar depression (35 percent of cases) or bipolar disorder (48 percent), based on 10-year follow-up after an index episode of depression (Geller et al., 2002; Geller & DelBello, 2003).

Central to the treatment of severe depression is not only reducing the suffering and disability experienced in the current episode but also anticipating these extraordinarily high rates of recurrence and addressing relapse prevention. Untreated depression in childhood and adolescence often leads to treatment-resistant depression in adulthood—a condition in which pharmacological and nonpharmacological interventions offer little relief from symptoms and disability.

# DIAGNOSTIC ISSUES

Although there are similarities between childhood-onset and adult-onset major depression, there are also notable differences. Use of the *Diagnostic and Statistical Manual of Mental Disorders, Fourth Edition* (*DSM-IV;* American Psychiatric Association, 2000) standard criteria for diagnosing major depression failed to accurately diagnose 76 percent of young children judged to be suffering from major depression (Luby et al., 2002). Little has changed in diagnostic criteria in *DSM-5* (American Psychiatric Association, 2013). For more diagnostic precision, Luby et al. recommend the modified diagnostic criteria listed in figure 2-A.

It is of interest that for many years, children with major depression were not believed to have vegetative signs (such as sleep or appetite disturbance), although these symptoms do occur in youngsters with major depression. Also, it is important to note that in children with depression, an irritable or anhedonic mood is almost as common as a sad or depressed mood. Fortunately, the symptom of anhedonia is often associated with depression and makes an accurate diagnosis of depression more likely. Irritability, on the other hand, may be attributed to other psychiatric conditions such as oppositional defiant disorder, attention-deficit/hyperactivity disorder, bipolar disorder, and others. Consequently, this increases the likelihood of an inaccurate diagnosis and treatment plan. See figure 2-B for a list of additional depressive symptoms.

## SYMPTOMS OF MAJOR DEPRESSION IN CHILDREN

Four of the following (as opposed to the five required for adults to be diagnosed with major depression):

- Depressed or irritable mood for more days than not
- Anhedonia (markedly diminished interest or pleasure in all or almost all activities, most days)
- Significant weight loss or gain (or failure to make expected weight gain)
- Insomnia or hypersomnia more days than not
- Psychomotor agitation or retardation
- Fatigue more days than not
- Feelings of worthlessness or excessive guilt
- Impaired concentration (often accompanied by a precipitous drop in grades)
- Recurrent thoughts of death or suicide

**Figure 2-A**

## ADDITIONAL DIAGNOSTIC SIGNS AND SYMPTOMS OF MAJOR DEPRESSION IN CHILDREN

**Most Common Symptoms**

- Irritability
- Social withdrawal
- Anhedonia
- Low self-esteem
- Themes of death, suicide, or self-destruction appearing in play
- Vegetative symptoms (such as sleep disturbance or poor appetite)

**Common Symptoms**

- School failure
- Loneliness
- Sadness
- Low energy

**Associated Signs and Symptoms**

- Vague, nonspecific physical complaints
- Running away from home
- Boredom
- Extreme sensitivity to rejection or failure
- Reckless behavior; acting out
- Difficulty with relationships
- Substance use or abuse

**Figure 2-B**

In almost half of prepubertal children with episodes of major depression, the first episode ultimately turns out to have been the earliest manifestation of bipolar illness. Of people with prepubertal bipolar disorder, 70 percent initially present with depression and, on average, have two to four depressive episodes prior to their first manic episode (Geller & DelBello, 2003). Thus the clinician, in addition to making a diagnosis of major depression, must also conduct a comprehensive evaluation to rule out potential bipolarity in all depressed children and teenagers. This is especially critical in light of the growing concern that the use of antidepressants may, in the long run, be risky in bipolar patients (potentially exacerbating a manic episode or causing cycle acceleration, a worsening of the disorder, discussed in chapter 3). The history and clinical features given in figure 2-C should alert the clinician to a higher risk of bipolar disorder. However, the best place to start when determining whether or not a child is suffering from unipolar or bipolar depression is to look at the family history, specifically the presence of bipolar disorder in the parents or siblings. Genetics play a key role in bipolar disorder.

Disruptive mood dysregulation disorder (DMDD) is a new diagnosis in *DSM-5.* It is marked by persistent irritability and episodes of temper outbursts. Severe, nonepisodic irritability has been seen as a manifestation of pediatric bipolar disorder by a number of researchers. This might account for some of the significant increases in bipolar disorder diagnoses in youth (American Psychiatric Association, 2013, p.157). One feature of DMDD that differs from most cases of bipolar disorder is that it is very persistent (i.e., not episodic, as are most cases of bipolar disorder). Longitudinal studies strongly indicate that years later, most people who suffered from DMDD do not go on to have bipolar disorder. The psychiatric problems seen later are primarily major depression and anxiety disorders. See figure 2-D for symptoms of DMDD.

## RED FLAGS FOR POSSIBLE BIPOLAR DISORDER

- Atypical depressive symptoms such as hypersomnia (excessive sleeping), severe fatigue, increased appetite, carbohydrate craving, and weight gain
- Seasonal (winter) depressions
- Psychotic symptoms (e.g., delusions)
- History of separation anxiety disorder
- History of attention-deficit/hyperactivity disorder (ADHD) or ADHD-like symptoms[1]
- Positive family history of bipolar disorder
- History of hypomania

**Figure 2-C**

1 Most children with a history of ADHD do not develop bipolar disorder, but some individuals with prepubertal-onset bipolar disorder do show a history of behaviors during infancy and early childhood that resemble ADHD. This topic will be addressed more extensively in chapters 3 and 6.

SYMPTOMS OF DISRUPTIVE MOOD DYSREGULATION DISORDER

**(also see American Psychiatric Association, 2013**)

• Frequent (3 or more a week) and severe temper outbursts, grossly out of proportion in intensity and duration

• Persistent (nearly every day) anger and irritability

• Symptoms have been present for 12 months or more

• Not diagnosed for the first time before age 6 or after age 18

• Absence of manic symptoms (and no history of manic symptoms)

**Figure 2-D**

# PSYCHOPHARMACOLOGY

## *Efficacy of Antidepressants*

Early case reports and clinical experience have shown that *very severely depressed, hospitalized* children and adolescents often respond to treatment with tricyclic antidepressants (Walkup, 2004). At the same time, tricyclics can have significant side effects, are very toxic in overdoses, and have been associated with six cases of sudden death in children (due to cardiac effects with the tricyclic desipramine). Additionally, in recent controlled studies, tricyclics have been found to be no more effective than placebos in the treatment of mild to moderate major depression (as mentioned earlier, severely ill children are not included in such studies). Thus, in this chapter, we will address only the newer (nontricyclic) antidepressants. For those interested in a more in-depth review of tricyclic antidepressants, see Gillman (2007).

To date, the double-blind, placebo-controlled studies of antidepressants in the treatment of major depression have been limited to selective serotonin reuptake inhibitors (SSRIs, such as Prozac and Zoloft) and, in one study, venlafaxine (although drugs such as bupropion [Wellbutrin] are in common use, and other classes of drugs are undergoing trials). Placebo responses in these child studies are higher than those seen in adult studies; thus, in order to be judged, from a statistical standpoint, significantly better than placebo, the drug must have a very high level of demonstrated efficacy and large enough sample sizes. The limited studies in this area of investigation reveal that SSRIs are much better tolerated than tricyclics and are significantly more effective than either placebos or tricyclics (Emslie & Mayes, 2001; Wagner et al., 2003; March et al., 2004; Whittington et al., 2004; Qin et al., 2014). Supporting the notions of greater efficacy and higher placebo effects, a recent meta-analysis that analyzed 6,500 patients across 36 studies with a variety of psychiatric conditions revealed that antidepressant therapy was more beneficial than placebo; however, the clinical effects were small and the effects of placebo were large when looking only at studies of depression. It was also noted in the study that those who were treated with antidepressants complained of greater side effects compared with those who took a placebo (Locher et al., 2017).

In contrast, a meta-analysis of studies by Jureidini et al. (2004) shows an effect size across six randomized, placebo-controlled studies of just 0.26. This is a very small effect size and *may* suggest that antidepressant efficacy is limited compared with placebo. On the other hand, it is important to note that most of the studies reviewed in this meta-analysis suffered from significant methodological flaws (Walkup, 2004). These studies were supported by pharmaceutical companies and done largely in response to an FDA incentive: "Companies could extend their patents for a drug for 6 months by testing it on children ... whether the trial demonstrated that the drug worked or not. There was, in other words, a powerful incentive to do the trials, but no incentive to do them well" (Mahler, 2004).

A federally funded program, Treatments for Adolescents with Depression Study (TADS), has addressed many of the methodological issues raised in other studies and provides further evidence supporting the use of antidepressants for childhood depression.

The sample included 432 adolescents (ages 12 to 17) suffering from major depression. The subjects were randomly assigned to one of four groups. At the completion of the 12 weeks of treatment, the percentages of positive responders were: placebo, 35 percent; cognitive behavioral therapy (CBT), 43 percent; fluoxetine (Prozac), 61 percent; and combination CBT and fluoxetine, 71 percent. Here, drug treatments were significantly more effective than placebo or psychotherapy alone. The effect sizes were 0.8 and 0.6 for the combination treatment and fluoxetine alone, respectively (Glass, 2004; March et al., 2004). Obviously, these results are promising and underscore the benefits of combining medication treatment with psychotherapy.

In evaluating high placebo response rates, which are common, it is very important to keep in mind that, although acute treatment-placebo responses in children are impressively high, no study has evaluated the ability of placebos to prevent breakthrough symptoms or to reduce episode recurrence. Currently available efficacy studies are limited in duration (8 to 18 weeks), and there is an absence of long-term follow-up. Typically positive placebo responses, if they occur, tend to be time limited. Owing to the highly recurrent nature of depression in youngsters, the issue of longer-term effects is crucial, although systematic data on this issue are lacking. In other words, the youngster may show a significant response to placebo in the early stages of a clinical study (and in clinical practice), but in many cases the depressive symptoms will return. Conversely, antidepressant medication may show similar or only slightly better effects than placebo, but the positive effects of the antidepressant will outlast those seen with placebo.

Two findings from these empirical studies and clinical experience appear to be important to note: (1) the time to onset of positive medication effects may be longer for children than for adults (with children, although symptomatic improvement may be noted within 4 weeks, in some instances an adequate trial of 8 to 12 weeks is required); and (2) a syndrome of apathy/amotivation or emotional disinhibition, sometimes seen in adults on longer-term SSRI and serotonin and norepinephrine reuptake inhibitor (SNRI) treatment, is more commonly encountered in children (Barnhart, Makela, & Latocha, 2004; Walkup, 2004).

## *An Overview of Antidepressant Medications*

Currently only one antidepressant, fluoxetine (Prozac, Sarafem), is approved by the FDA for the treatment of major depression in children (ages 8 and older); however, as mentioned in chapter 1, many antidepressants are in widespread off-label use. Antidepressants are commonly listed in most psychopharmacology textbooks according to the neurotransmitters they target: SSRIs, NRIs (norepinephrine reuptake inhibitors), SNRIs, NDRIs (norepinephrine and dopamine reuptake inhibitors [Wellbutrin]), and atypical antidepressants (trazodone, vortioxetine, and mirtazapine). Antidepressant medications are listed by class, names, recommended starting doses, and typical daily doses in figure 2-E, and common side effects are listed in figure 2-F.

| ANTIDEPRESSANT MEDICATIONS | | | | |
|---|---|---|---|---|
| **Generic Name** | **Brand Name** | **Starting Dose (mg)** | **Daily Dose (mg)** | **Daily Dose (Weight[2] Adjusted, mg/kg[2])** |
| **SSRI** | | | | |
| Fluoxetine | Prozac,<br>Sarafem | C[1]: 5<br>A[1]: 10 | 5–40<br>10–60 | 0.25–0.75 |
| Sertraline | Zoloft | C: 25<br>A: 50 | 25–200<br>50–200 | 1.5–3.0 |
| Paroxetine | Paxil | C: 5<br>A: 10 | 10–30<br>20–50 | 0.25–0.75 |
| Citalopram | Celexa | C: 10<br>A: 10 | 10–40<br>10–40 | 0.25–0.75 |
| Escitalopram | Lexapro | C: 5<br>A: 5 | 5–20<br>5–20 | 0.125–0.375 |
| Fluvoxamine | Luvox | C: 25<br>A: 25–50 | 25–200<br>50–200 | 1.5–4.5 |
| **SNRI** | | | | |
| Venlafaxine XR | Effexor XR | C: 12.5<br>A: 25–37.5 | 12.5–37.5<br>25–75+ | 1–2 |
| Desvenla-faxine | Pristiq | C: Not established<br>A: 50 | Not established<br>50–300 | Not established |
| Duloxetine | Cymbalta | C: Not established<br>A: 10 | Not established<br>20–80 | 1 |
| Levomilnaci-pran | Fetzima | C: Not established<br>A: 20 | Not established | 1<br><br>40–120 |

| | | | | |
|---|---|---|---|---|
| **NRI** | | | | |
| Atomoxetine | Strattera | C: 10<br>A: 40 | 10–60<br>40–100 | 1.2–1.8 |
| **NDRI** | | | | |
| Bupropion SR | Wellbutrin SR | C: 100<br>A: 100 | 50–150<br>150–300 | 3–6 |
| **Atypical** | | | | |
| Mirtazapine | Remeron | C: 7.5<br>A: 15 | 15–30<br>15–45 | Not established |
| Trazodone[3] | Desyrel | C: 25<br>A: 50 | 25–75<br>25–100 | 1–3 |
| Vortioxetine | Brintellix | C: Not established<br>A: 10 | Not established<br>10–20 | Not established |
| Vilazodone[4] | Viibryd | C: Not established<br>A: 10 | Not established<br>10–40 | Not established |

1 C: prepubertal children; A: adolescents/adults

2 To convert pounds to kilograms, divide number of pounds by 2.2.

3 Trazodone is technically an antidepressant but has limited efficacy in treating depression. However, it is often used as a non-habit-forming medication for the treatment of initial insomnia. The doses in the chart are those used to treat insomnia.

4 Efficacy, dosing, and safety data have not been established for Vilazodone in young children or adolescents. It is not currently recommended for use in individuals under the age of 18.

Figure 2-E

| COMMON SIDE EFFECTS OF ANTIDEPRESSANTS | | | | | |
|---|---|---|---|---|---|
| **Medication** | **Activation**[1] | **Sedation** | **Nausea** | **Sexual Dysfunction**[2] | **Weight Gain** |
| **SSRI** | | | | | |
| Fluoxetine | +++ | +/0 | + | ++ | 3 |
| Sertraline | ++ | +/0 | ++ | ++ | 3 |
| Paroxetine | + | ++ | + | ++ | 3 |
| Citalopram | + | +/0 | + | ++ | 3 |
| Escitalopram | + | +/0 | + | ++ | 3 |
| Fluvoxamine | +/0 | ++ | ++ | ++ | 3 |
| **SNRI** | | | | | |
| Venlafaxine | + | + | + | ++ | 3 |
| Desvenlafaxine | + | + | + | ++ | 3 |
| Duloxetine | + | + | ++ | + | 4 |
| Levomilnacipran | + | + | ++ | + | 4 |
| **NRI** | | | | | |
| Atomoxetine | + | ++ | +/0 | 0 | 0 |
| **NDRI** | | | | | |
| Bupropion | ++ | 0 | + | 0 | 0 |

| | | | | | |
|---|---|---|---|---|---|
| **Atypical** | | | | | |
| Mirtazapine | +/0 | ++ | 0 | ++ | +++ |
| Trazodone[5] | 0 | +++ | 0 | 0 | 0 |
| Vortioxetine | + | + | + | + | 3 |
| Vilazodone[6] | + | + | ++ | + | 3 |

Key: +++: substantial side effects; ++: moderate side effects; +: mild side effects; +/0: possible side effects; 0: none

1 This is an acute side effect occurring within a few hours of the first dose of the medication or when there is a dosage increase; includes anxiety and insomnia that can continue during the first two weeks of treatment but often subsides thereafter.

2 Primarily inorgasmia, reported by approximately 25 to 30 percent of patients; can be associated with all SSRIs, venlafaxine, desvenlafaxine, and duloxetine.

3 Acute weight gain is rare. A small percentage (possibly 10 percent) of patients may experience weight gain after being on the medication for 12 months or more.

4 Not yet determined.

5 The low incidence of side effects (except sedation) assumes the use of low doses, e.g., 25–50 mg (see figure 2-D).

6 Data are limited for vilazodone as it relates to the treatment of depression with children and adolescents.

Figure 2-F

In addition to prescription antidepressants, two over-the-counter products have demonstrated some efficacy in treating depression: Saint-John's-wort and SAM-e. Although there are a number of outcome studies of these drugs in the treatment of adults with depression, no such studies have been conducted with children or adolescents, and thus they should be considered to be experimental. It should be noted that Saint-John's-wort has been associated with significant effects on liver metabolism and can adversely interact with other medications, including birth control pills, which it may render ineffective.

## *Guidelines for the Pharmacological Treatment of Depression*

Treatment is started with low doses during the first week (see figure 2-D) and then, if tolerated, gradually increased. A low starting dose is important because approximately 5 percent of children have a condition referred to as "2D6 hypometabolism." This condition causes an inadequate first-pass metabolism of some drugs, including antidepressants, resulting in high levels of the drug in the bloodstream and, thus, very significant side effects (2D6 is a liver enzyme that is responsible for metabolizing a number of antidepressants and other drugs). Were these children to be started on higher doses, the initial side effects could be overwhelming.

One of the most common problems in initiating treatment is activation, an acute-onset side effect that may occur within a few hours of taking the first dose of a drug or when dosages are increased. Patients experiencing activation present with anxiety, initial insomnia (trouble falling asleep), and sometimes agitation. It is important to note that this is different from switching, which occurs when an antidepressant provokes the emergence of mania or hypomania in a person with bipolar disorder. Switching generally does not occur until the medication has been taken for two or more weeks (thus, the main differential features of activation versus switching are the time of onset, and activation being primarily anxiety whereas switching includes all symptoms of mania [see chapter 3]).

Because activation can be unpleasant, when parents see it, they may not only stop the medication but also become afraid of and pessimistic about psychiatric drug treatment in general. Thus, parents need to be advised that activation can happen and, if it does, to contact the doctor right away. Clinicians can also co-prescribe a low dose of a minor tranquilizer (such as lorazepam [Ativan], 0.125mg) and instruct the parents to give it to their child if signs of activation appear. Fortunately, activation generally subsides within one to two weeks. By the end of the first month of treatment, tranquilizers are usually no longer necessary. The best way to avoid the specific antidepressant side effect of activation is to start with a low dose of the medication and increase it slowly as tolerated. If the initial dose does not lead to activation, but appears upon a dose increase, the child can revert back to the original dose and increase the medication more slowly the second time. This can be done by cutting the pill in half or quarters, pouring a portion of the contents of a capsule into a beverage or food, or administering the medication every other day. However, these techniques do not work for all medications, and specific administration instructions like these should come directly from the prescribing clinician.

The general rule of thumb is to start with a low dose, as mentioned previously, and then increase the dose while carefully watching for signs of either a clinical response or the emergence of side effects (which would suggest that the dose is too high). There are no well-established guidelines for how long to wait between dosage adjustments, although it is common practice to treat for 1 month to 6 weeks and then to increase the dose if there has been no sign of clinical improvement (generally this is a better first-step strategy than switching to a different drug or adding a second medication). Please also keep in mind that some children are late responders, and there is some positive yield by continuing to treat for a number of weeks until clinical improvement is noted.

If a positive clinical response occurs, then how long does continuation treatment last? The answer to this question has not been clearly determined in efficacy studies. It is well known that in adults and older adolescents, it is very important to continue treatment with an antidepressant at the *same dose* for a minimum of 6 months after symptomatic improvement, followed then by gradual discontinuation. If the person has had a previous depressive episode, treatment may need to last 9 to 12 months (several past episodes may necessitate indefinite treatment). This guideline has often been adopted in the treatment of children as well, despite the absence of empirical support for this strategy.

The clinician should be alert to the possible development of two late-onset side effects that can be seen in some patients treated with antidepressants (this is the case for all antidepressants except bupropion [Wellbutrin]): (1) apathy and emotional blunting, and (2) emotional disinhibition, both apparently due to the downstream effect of serotonin on the dopamine neurotransmitter system in the frontal lobes (Barnhart et al., 2004). These often-unrecognized side effects completely subside with discontinuation of medication or may respond favorably to the coadministration of bupropion (which activates the dopamine neurotransmitter system).

## Antidepressants and Suicidality

The media have given a good deal of attention to the potential risks of antidepressants and their connection to increased suicidality (especially in children and adolescents). The matter was initially brought up by a study in England (referred to in Aursnes, Tvete, Gaasemyr, & Natvig, 2005) that raised concerns about increased suicidality in young patients treated with the antidepressant Paxil (paroxetine). In this study, which included 1,300 patients, Paxil was compared with placebo, and increased suicidality was reported in 1.2 percent of placebo-and 3.4 percent of Paxil-treated subjects. Although this difference is statistically significant, it is important to note that there were no actual suicides in this group of youngsters, and that a number of suicidal "events" occurred in the Paxil group when the children *stopped* taking the medication.

Also, in trying to understand and address this issue, we face one significant problem: the concept of suicidality has been very loosely defined in this and other studies. In most cases it includes reports of increased thoughts about suicide, suicidal gestures, and non-lethal-intent self-mutilation (as is often seen in people with borderline personality disorder or in people with a history of severe neglect). In one instance, even a report of a child slapping herself qualified as a suicide attempt (Brown University, 2004). Of course, actual suicides and lethal attempts are also included under this umbrella of suicidality.

Concerns regarding increased suicidality have had a significant impact on both the prescribing of antidepressants and parental fears about the use of these drugs. The FDA has also responded to concerns about increased suicidality by requiring drug companies to issue warnings about the use of these drugs with younger clients, and initiated a study in 2007 to investigate the data—an examination of a database of 4,400 teenagers treated with antidepressants. The results were consistent with the earlier findings; 4 out of 100 children and adolescents taking an antidepressant experienced suicidal thoughts or behavior compared with 2 out of 100 taking a placebo. No suicides occurred in either group. It is interesting to note that in these large groups of children and adolescents treated with SSRIs, there have been no suicides. A 2012 study followed 9,185 patients being treated with antidepressants; included were four randomized, placebo-controlled trials with 708 children and adolescents treated with Prozac. This review found reduced suicidality in adults and geriatric patients and no evidence of increased suicidal risk in youth (Gibbons, Brown, Hur, Davis, & Mann, 2012).

Even though the likelihood of increased suicidality may be low in large group studies, the clinician must be on the lookout for the emergence of suicidal tendencies in all patients who suffer from major depression. It is certainly possible that in some cases, drugs can contribute to this problem. The following may account for increased suicidality seen in some individuals treated with antidepressants:

- Activation and akathisia (increased restlessness) may add to a general sense of emotional discomfort.
- Antidepressants can provoke mixed (dysphoric) mania in some youngsters who, in fact, have bipolar disorder. (See chapter 3.)
- Increased energy may occur before a decrease in depressive mood (giving the person the energy to carry out a suicide attempt).
- Noncompliance.

Noncompliance (patient-or parent-initiated discontinuation) can result in two common, problematic results that might account for increased suicidality: antidepressant withdrawal symptoms (see Medication Discontinuation later in this chapter) and/or the loss of what had been a positive antidepressant effect, plunging the patient back into depression.

What is clear is that untreated major depression carries significant risk of suicide. Treatment with antidepressants takes several weeks before the first signs of clinical improvement appear, and depression can worsen during this start-up period of treatment. In evaluating these kinds of concerns, we must always differentiate between media hype and scientific data. Refer parents who may be interested in this issue to the National Institute of Mental Health (NIMH) website (http://www.nimh.nih.gov).

## *Treatment of Depressive Subtypes*

There are several nonblinded studies showing the effectiveness of antidepressants in the treatment of persistent depressive disorder (dysthymia) in children (Nobile, Cataldo, Marino, & Molteni, 2003). Treating dysthymia is important since without treatment it generally lasts for at least

3 to 4 years, with substantial negative effects on psychosocial functioning and development. Additionally, many if not most children with dysthymia eventually develop major depression. It is unclear whether early treatment of dysthymia can prevent major depression later, although professionals speculate that it can. Obviously, further study is needed to confirm the efficacy of antidepressants in treating dysthymia.

SSRIs are effective agents for treating premenstrual dysphoric disorder (PMDD). (Note that the nonserotonin antidepressants such as NRIs and NDRIs are not effective in treating PMDD.) Unlike patients being treated for other depressive disorders, PMDD patients often have an acute positive response to treatment with SSRIs, sometimes showing symptomatic improvement several hours after taking the first dose. Additionally, generally patients need only take the medication for the period of time that they typically experience emotional symptoms, perhaps only a few days every month, thus allowing them to avoid longer-term side effects.

Many severe types of major depression in young people present with psychotic symptoms. Often, psychotic symptoms are not as easy to observe in people with mood disorders as they are in patients with schizophrenia or drug-induced psychosis. Many very depressed youngsters harbor delusional thoughts (for example, "I always have a fever even though my parents say I don't, and the fever is destroying my brain"; "I'm the worst person in the world ... even the president hates me"; "Other kids are spraying chemicals on my backpack that are making me fail in school"; a teenager: "My car is bugged ... some kids hate me, and they are doing this to make me think that I am going crazy") but keep these thoughts to themselves, and clinicians may treat them for months before appreciating the psychotic aspect of the disorder. Thus it is very important to carefully assess for the presence of these lessobvious signs of psychosis. Psychotic symptoms necessitate the use of antipsychotic medications (in conjunction with antidepressants) or the use of electroconvulsive therapy (ECT).

Additionally, the presence of psychotic symptoms should strongly increase one's index of suspicion that the patient has bipolar disorder (see chapter 3).

## *Medication Discontinuation*

Discontinuation withdrawal symptoms have been well documented. These symptoms, which occur with abrupt discontinuation, generally include nausea, body aches, nervousness, insomnia, a peculiar "electrical shock" sensation experienced periodically, and generalized body aches like those that come with the flu. There have been reports of increased suicidality upon rapid discontinuation, possibly due to one or both of the following factors: either the medication was controlling the depression and, with its discontinuation, it is no longer having this effect, or the distress caused by withdrawal symptoms has provoked the emergence of suicidal feelings. Severe withdrawal symptoms are most likely to be seen in connection with two drugs (both of which have short half-lives): Paxil and Effexor. Withdrawal symptoms can occur with the discontinuation of most other antidepressants as well, with the exception of Prozac (with which it occurs very rarely, due to its long half-life). Withdrawal symptoms can generally be avoided if the medication is gradually discontinued over a period of several weeks.

## *Relapse Prevention*

Adults experiencing a third episode of major depression are best treated by ongoing, chronic antidepressant therapy to reduce the likelihood of recurrence. As noted earlier, many if not most children experiencing a major depression will have recurrences. However, there are inadequate data to support chronic use of antidepressants with youngsters. Thus, until more research is available to address this issue, it is probably prudent to gradually discontinue medications after 6 months of asymptomatic status (as noted above) and educate the patient and his or her parents to watch for signs of possible recurrence. If these signs are spotted, parents should seek treatment as soon as possible.

# CHAPTER 3

# Bipolar Disorder

For adolescents, the prevalence of bipolar disorder, or cyclothymia, is approximately 1 percent (and 5 to 6 percent for subsyndromal symptoms) (Lewinsohn, Klein, & Seeley, 1995, 2000; Costello et al., 2002) with some estimates of the former being as high as 3 percent (Merikangas et al., 2010). Many cases of bipolar disorder have their onset in childhood or adolescence—prepubertal children: 15 percent; teenagers up to the age of 18: 35 percent; and adults: 50 percent (STEP-BD Program, 2008). For many patients, manic symptoms begin during mid-adolescence.

The prevalence of bipolar disorder in young children has not been established due to lack of large-scale epidemiological studies. There is a growing recognition that bipolar disorder does affect children in some cases. However, controversy concerning the prepubertal diagnosis of bipolar disorder remains. Areas of debate include the accurate establishment of the age of onset, implications of comorbid conditions, atypical presentations, definition of symptom criteria, and the impact that drug company–sponsored research has had on estimates of prevalence.

## Escalation of Bipolar Disorder Diagnoses

Since the mid-1990s, the diagnosis of bipolar disorder has increased significantly: two-fold among adults, four-fold among adolescents, and forty-fold with children (Moreno et al., 2007)! There is general agreement among mood-disorder experts that (especially with children) this has become the diagnosis du jour and most of these children do not have true bipolar disorder. (It is not unlike the explosion of ADHD diagnoses over the past two decades in which prevalence estimates have nearly doubled.) Mood instability is a hallmark symptom of many psychiatric disorders and does not automatically imply a diagnosis of bipolar disorder. To a degree, it is also a byproduct of normal maturation.

Common disorders that present with mood instability include the following:

- Diffuse brain damage (e.g., due to fetal alcohol exposure, traumatic brain injuries)
- Anxiety disorders
- Post-traumatic stress disorder
- Situational stress
- Reactive attachment disorders
- Agitated, unipolar depression
- Impaired affect regulation as a consequence of severe early abuse or neglect
- Psychotic disorders (e.g., schizophrenia)
- Some neurodevelopmental disorders
- Substance use disorder (including caffeine and nicotine)

Misdiagnosis is not just an academic issue. Drugs that are used to treat bipolar disorder have significant adverse effects and expose patients to side effects that range from mild to potentially life-threatening.

Why such an increase in bipolar diagnoses? Some have suggested the following: pharmaceutical company marketing (especially aimed at increasing sales of antipsychotics); parents' desire to have their children diagnosed with a "biochemical" disorder, a shame-free biological explanation with a medication "quick fix"; or diagnostic "up-coding"—the practice of giving a patient a more severe diagnosis (i.e., not what the patient actually has) in order to have insurance companies pay for the treatment (Carlat, 2006).

What is clear are four issues:

1. It is likely that more youngsters with the actual disorder *are* being identified and treated.

2. At the same time, bipolar disorder is misdiagnosed in youth (this is likely one of the main reasons that bipolar disorder is overdiagnosed).

3. There is controversy and confusion among clinicians and researchers regarding specific criteria

for making a bipolar diagnosis in children.

4. Standard treatments that have a positive track record with adults and older adolescents are not nearly as effective with prepubertal children.

# DIAGNOSTIC ISSUES

The diagnosis of early-onset bipolar disorder is often difficult to establish, especially in young children. The *DSM-5* (American Psychiatric Association, 2013) diagnostic criteria are essentially the same for children, adolescents, and adults. However, the symptom presentation in young patients may not be clearly recognizable or may overlap with those of other disorders. Nottelmann, Biederman, Birmaher, Carlson, et al. (2001) estimate that only 40 percent of prepubertal patients referred to clinics for evaluation of bipolar disorder meet *DSM* criteria for bipolar I or bipolar II disorder. Several expert consensus groups are seeking to provide desperately needed diagnostic clarity, including developmentally appropriate criteria and instruments, with high interrater reliability and validity. A brief review of various bipolar disorder criteria is provided below.

For a diagnosis of bipolar I, the patient must have had at least one manic or mixed episode, characterized by abnormally elevated or irritable mood, of at least one week in duration (or less if hospitalization was required). Often patients have a history of one or more major depressive episodes. Functional impairment will be evident, as well as three or four additional symptoms from the following list:

- Grandiosity. In children this often presents as an overestimation of one's own abilities, which is a change from the child's normal behavior. This is qualitatively different from the overconfidence and assuredness that come from immaturity and inexperience associated with adolescence.
- Elevated or expansive mood. In children this often presents as significantly inappropriate or exaggerated silliness. The "significantly inappropriate or

exaggerated silliness" aspect of the behavior can be difficult to distinguish from baseline due to incredible individual variability in personality, style, and temperament of children.

- Decreased need for sleep (versus forcing oneself to avoid sleep for more pleasurable activities such as play or watching television).
- Flight of ideas
- Distractibility
- Pressured speech
- Increased activity. In children this symptom may manifest in taking on too many tasks or unrealistic projects. Also it may present as inappropriate sexual behavior. (Note that before assuming that inappropriate sexual behavior is a symptom of bipolar disorder, the possibility of sexual abuse history must be ruled out.)
- Risk-taking behavior

A mixed episode is defined as at least a 1-week period during which the criteria for both a manic episode and a depressive episode (except duration) are met. Mixed episodes, which are more prevalent among young patients, are characterized by the following:

- Hospitalization, psychotic features, significant impairment in academic or social functioning
- Dysphoria
- Disorganized thinking or behavior
- Extreme irritability

Bipolar II is diagnosed following at least one hypomanic episode and one depressive episode. Hypomania is a marked, observable, uncharacteristic elevation in mood, lasting at least 4 days, plus three or four of the symptoms listed above. There is no functional impairment or hospitalization.

Some researchers and clinicians propose modified diagnostic criteria for juvenile-onset bipolar disorder. For example, Liebenluft, Charney, Towbin, Bhangoo, & Pine (2003) suggest four bipolarity categories for children, with the following definitions:

1. Meets full *DSM* criteria for hypomania or mania, including duration, and displays classic elevated mood or grandiosity
2. Meets the *DSM* symptom criteria for hypomania or mania, but not

duration criteria, with hypomanic episodes lasting two to three days in length

3. Meets duration criteria, but episodes are characterized by irritability, not euphoria
4. Mood disorder, NOS (not otherwise specified): predominant symptoms are irritability and hyperarousal (not euphoria), which are chronic, not episodic

There are advantages to adopting the expanded-spectrum approach, including earlier diagnosis and treatment. However, many experts recommend using caution when deviating from *DSM* criteria, because the disadvantages are misdiagnosis and inappropriate treatments, which in some cases may worsen the clinical course or put the child at risk for potentially life-threatening consequences.

Papolos and Papolos (2007) and Coyle et al. (2003) have attempted to address the diagnostic complexities by summarizing how the signs and symptoms of early-onset bipolar disorder may differ from those of the disorder in adults. (See below and note that such symptoms are quite similar to disruptive mood dysregulation disorder, discussed in chapter 2).

## *SIGNS AND SYMPTOMS OF EARLY-ONSET MANIA*

- Chronic, not episodic
- Mixed states commonly occur with marked dysphoria and irritability
- Severe oppositional behavior
- Ultrarapid cycling
- Explosive outbursts or rage episodes

Carlson, Bromet, & Sievers (2000) provide a useful analysis of earlyversus adult-onset psychotic mania. In this study, early-onset subjects were aged 15 to 20 years, and adult subjects were defined as over age 30. A higher number of early-onset subjects

- were male
- had a history of childhood behavior disorders
- abused substances
- displayed paranoia
- experienced less-frequent episode remissions during 24-month follow-up

Finally, youth who suffer from bipolar disorder often have a strong family history of bipolar disorder. In fact, the heritability of bipolar disorder based on twin studies is believed to be around 60 to 80 percent, although some studies report slightly lower rates (Smoller & Finn, 2003; Wray & Gottesman, 2012). It is important to explore family history looking for the following in blood relatives: psychiatric hospitalizations, past use of psychotropic medication, severe alcohol abuse, suicide attempts and suicides, multiple marriages, persistent financial and legal problems, and starting numerous new jobs. The bottom line is that there is a strong likelihood of bipolar disorder occurring in children whose parents have bipolar disorder.

## Bipolar Disorder and Attention-Deficit/Hyperactivity Disorder (ADHD): Differential Diagnosis

Comorbid conditions include ADHD, anxiety disorders, oppositional defiant disorder, learning disorders, and substance abuse. Determining the bipolar–ADHD boundary in children poses particular diagnostic difficulties and is one of the most challenging differential diagnoses to make. As shown in figure 3-A, the overlap between symptoms of ADHD and bipolar disorder is significant.

## SYMPTOMATIC SIMILARITIES: ADHD AND CHILDHOOD-ONSET MANIA

- Irritability
- Inattention
- Hyperactivity
- Impulsivity
- High level of energy
- Pressured speech
- Symptoms are chronic and nonepisodic

**Figure 3-A**

Figure 3-B lists clinical features and other factors that help to differentiate ADHD from bipolar illnesses.

## DIFFERENTIATING BIPOLAR DISORDER FROM ADHD

**Symptoms Common to Bipolar Disorder but Very Rare With ADHD** [2]

- Decreased need for sleep without daytime fatigue
- Intense, prolonged rage attacks (lasting 2 to 4 hours)
- Hypersexuality
- Flight of ideas
- Morbid nightmares[3]
- Psychotic symptoms
- Family history of obvious bipolar disorder or one or more of the following in blood relatives:
  * Suicide or repeated suicide attempts
  * Severe alcohol or drug abuse
  * Multiple marriages
  * Persistent financial and legal problems
  * Tendency to start numerous businesses
- Hyperthymia (a form of chronic hypomania characterized by high

2 Geller & DelBello, 2003, pp.25–50.

3 Popper, 2004.

energy and productivity, gregariousness, impulsive behavior, and decreased need for sleep)

**Figure 3-B**

**Bipolar Disorder and ADHD: Comorbidity**

The association between early-onset bipolar disorder and ADHD continues to be a topic of considerable debate. The major discussion points are summarized below:

- Bipolar and ADHD may represent distinct disease entities.
- In some children with ADHD, the ADHD may be a prodrome of bipolar disorder. (Most children with ADHD do not go on to develop bipolar illness, and most bipolar patients do not have early ADHD-like symptoms. Thus there may be a subtype of bipolar illness that simply presents with early signs that mimic ADHD.)
- Childhood-onset bipolar disorder may be related to other bipolar-spectrum conditions but

represent a particular subtype of mood disorder (in other words, it is in some ways different from adult-onset bipolar conditions).

- Comorbid early-onset bipolar disorder and ADHD may constitute a distinct and particularly serious syndrome.

The actual rate of juvenile-onset bipolar disorder and ADHD comorbidity is not firmly established. The reported rate of co-occurrence is high: up to 80 percent for children and 30 percent for adolescents. However, many of the studies have methodological limitations. For example, Geller, Sun, Luby, Frazier, & Williams (1995) examined only rapid-cycling and mixed-episode patients. Findings reported by Wozniak, Biederman, Mundy, Mennin, & Faraone (1995) were based on a family-focused pilot study. Small sample sizes and retrospective design are limitations found in many studies. Sachs, Baldassano, Truman, & Guille (2000) advise cautious interpretation of results based on retrospective data collection from adults about their childhood symptoms. As mentioned previously, *although symptom overlap does occur,* most children with ADHD do not develop bipolar disorder later in life, and most bipolar patients do not have a history of fully diagnosed ADHD.

The idea that ADHD is a poorly defined subtype of bipolar disorder is not far-fetched. Stahl (2013) discusses in chapter 6 of his seminal text, *Stahl's Essential Psychopharmacology: Neuroscientific Basis and Practical Applications, Fourth Edition,* the notion that many patients present with symptoms that do not fit neatly within the current *DSM-5* bipolar disorder nomenclature. He discusses nine different subtypes of bipolar disorder with many more potential subtype possibilities.

Many critical questions remain unanswered. Are the comorbidities actual? Are the co-occurrence rates explained by the symptom overlap between the two disorders? Do the comorbidities represent a progressive or prodromal syndrome? Why is there a disparity in comorbidity rates (higher comorbidity when the primary diagnosis is bipolar disorder and lower rates when the primary diagnosis is ADHD)? Does treatment history contribute to comorbidity (for example, stimulant-induced mania)? Experts raise these questions and acknowledge the inherent limitations in the design and execution of existing research studies, categorically emphasizing the pressing need to establish diagnostic clarity.

### Bipolar Disorder and Anxiety Disorders

The clinician is faced with challenges when diagnosing and treating comorbid bipolar disorder and anxiety disorders. The family-genetic findings of Wozniak, Biederman, Monuteaux, Richards, & Faraone (2002) raise questions regarding whether bipolar–anxiety disorder comorbidity is a distinct clinical entity and to what degree anxiety may be a precursor of early-onset bipolar disorder.

Results of a study reported by Masi et al. (2004) point to earlier obsessive-compulsive disorder (OCD) onset and more severe OCD symptomatology in adolescent patients with comorbid bipolar disorder and OCD.

Findings of Birmaher et al. (2002) addressed the occurrence and severity of comorbid bipolar disorder and panic disorder. The presence of either panic disorder or bipolar disorder increased the likelihood of co-occurrence of the other. Psychotic symptoms and suicidal ideation were more frequent in youths with bipolar disorder and panic disorder than in patients with other comorbid mood (non-bipolar) and anxiety (non-panic) disorders.

Because of the risk of inducing mania, hypomania, or cycle acceleration, special attention must be paid to medication when treating comorbid bipolar and anxiety disorders. Antidepressants are a common treatment for some anxiety disorders, and the potential risks of using these medications when comorbid bipolar disorder is present must be considered. This is particularly true for medications with strong serotonergic and adrenergic properties and when treating OCD. Successful management of OCD symptoms typically requires higher doses of serotonergic medication, and activation of mania or hypomania appears to be dose dependent.

**Bipolar Disorder and Other Comorbidities**

Differentiating bipolar disorder from major depression is of critical importance, because 70 percent of cases of early-onset bipolar illness first become manifest in an episode of major depression. See chapter 2 for a discussion of the differentiation of major depression from bipolar disorder. As mentioned above, a potential consequence of misdiagnosing bipolar disorder as major depression, and treating with an antidepressant, is the triggering of a manic or hypomanic episode. Additionally, mood instability would persist due to the absence of a mood stabilizer, leading to further decompensation and potential harm to self or others.

In older adolescents, the distinction between bipolar disorder and schizophrenia sometimes presents a diagnostic challenge, especially with a first episode of psychotic mania. Because psychotic symptoms and anxiety are relatively common with bipolar onset prior to age 18, the differential diagnosis can be difficult. Misdiagnosing bipolar disorder as schizophrenia may result in the omission of a mood stabilizer from the medication regimen, which would not be beneficial to the patient. However, this concern has lessened over recent years as atypical antipsychotics, or what are sometimes referred to as second-generation antipsychotics (e.g., quetiapine, olanzapine, lurasidone), have been shown to be effective mood stabilizers in addition to controlling positive and negative symptoms of psychosis.

**Genes, Family Studies, and Genetic Risks**

Heritability of bipolar disorder has been demonstrated in familial, twin, and adoption studies (Tsuang & Faraone, 1990; Wray & Gottesman, 2012). Both genetic and environmental factors are presumed to be important. While no twin or adoption studies specific to pediatric bipolar disorder have been conducted to our knowledge, family studies demonstrate a strong familial component. Though genetic linkage studies are not conclusive, several chromosomes have been investigated. However, no consistent pattern of abnormal genes has been found in individuals with bipolar disorder. It is very likely that the neurobiological aspects of bipolar disorder are caused by a complex multitude of genes rather than one specific genetic abnormality. Epigenetics (environmental impact on gene expression) also may play a role (Stahl, 2013).

The relative risk of a child developing bipolar disorder if one parent has bipolar disorder is approximately 25 percent. Parents who have bipolar disorder are understandably concerned about the possibility that their child may develop the disorder. In these higher-risk children, the following are recommended: regular exercise, the use of omega-3 fatty acids (daily dose: 1,000mg of EPA, or eicosapentaenoic acid, which is one version of omega-3 fatty acids derived from fish oil; see chapter 9 for a discussion of over-the-counter products, such as omega-3 fatty acids), careful attention to sleeping habits, limiting exposure to highly stressful events, ensuring adequate amounts of sleep per night, and alertness to any early signs of behavioral changes or mood instability that might signal the onset of a first bipolar episode (DelBello, 2013).

# PSYCHOPHARMACOLOGY

## *Mood Stabilizers*

Pharmacotherapy is the mainstay of treatment of bipolar disorder. This section covers the three commonly used and studied mood stabilizers—lithium, divalproex (Depakote), and carbamazepine (Tegretol, Equetro)—as well as lamotrigine (Lamictal) oxcarbazepine (Trileptal), topiramate (Topamax), and atypical antipsychotics.

### LITHIUM

Lithium (Lithonate, Lithobid, Eskalith) is an established mood stabilizer, with 50-to 80-percent response rates for bipolar I disorder in adults and adolescents. However, positive outcomes with lithium in preadolescent bipolar patients are considerably lower. Some studies show that in this group of children, lithium (used alone) may be no more effective than placebo. Lithium is approved by the FDA for use in children 12 to 18 years of age. In adolescents, lithium is a first-line agent indicated for bipolar mania, bipolar depression, and prophylaxis. It has some efficacy in treating childhood-onset bipolar disorder if combined with Depakote or antipsychotic medications. The mechanism of action is unknown, but lithium has effects on multiple central nervous system components. Current research focuses on lithium's ability to stabilize neurochemical systems and its neuroprotective effects. Despite the efficacy of lithium, dosing requirements, side effects, and monitoring parameters may limit its use in pediatric patients.

Lithium is prescribed based on dosing recommendations, symptom response, and ongoing testing of blood levels. Lithium demonstrates a narrow therapeutic index—the therapeutic dose is very close to the toxic dose. Therefore, blood tests are required, which may limit use in pediatric patients. The onset of action of lithium is 5 to 14 days, although full symptom resolution may take up to several months. There are several formulations of lithium, including slow release and liquid versions.

Lithium has unique features in its ability to significantly reduce suicide. This is important since bipolar disorder is associated with very high suicide rates. It is important to note, however, that lithium is very toxic, and even small overdoses, whether intentional or accidental, can cause death (and there is no antidote). Thus, if pediatric bipolar patients are in a depressive or mixed-manic episode (when suicidal behaviors are common), lithium can be tricky to use because of the risk of overdose unless carefully monitored by parents. Once patients are stabilized or out of acute suicidal risk, however, lithium can be enormously important in further reducing that risk.

The side effects of lithium occur along a continuum, ranging from benign and transient to fatal. Common side effects include increased thirst, increased urination, nausea, vomiting, diarrhea, headache, cognitive slowing, tremor, weight gain, and worsening of acne. More serious, although less common, effects are changes in kidney function, hypothyroidism, cardiac conduction abnormalities, and increased white blood cell count. Lithium requires ongoing medical monitoring (blood tests) to measure lithium levels as well as tests of kidney and thyroid functioning. Frequent blood draws may make this a difficult treatment for some children. If a patient has been treated with lithium for several months, and the decision to stop treatment is being considered, caution is warranted. Suicide risk increases significantly with discontinuation.

## *Anticonvulsant Medications*

Divalproex and carbamazepine are anticonvulsant medications that have demonstrated efficacy in the treatment of bipolar disorder. Both of these agents are widely used to treat seizure disorders in pediatric patients. Lamotrigine, oxcarbazepine, and topiramate are less widely prescribed, both as anticonvulsants and as mood stabilizers. The mechanism of action of anticonvulsants in bipolar disorder is unknown. Among the properties of anticonvulsants are stabilization of cell membrane ion channels, potentiation of the inhibitory neurotransmitter GABA, and inhibition of the excitatory neurotransmitter glutamate. In addition, several anticonvulsants demonstrate neuroprotective properties, as does lithium.

**DIVALPROEX (DEPAKOTE)**

Divalproex is a first-line agent for mania and considered to be the preferred drug for mixed episodes in adults and adolescents. Opinions differ on whether it is the preferred drug for rapid cycling. Divalproex is FDA approved for bipolar mania in adults. Common side effects are nausea, vomiting, drowsiness, and weight gain. Less common, but more serious, are liver damage, pancreatitis, tremor, hair loss, blood clotting disorders, and polycystic ovary disease. Routine blood-level monitoring is required for divalproex, utilizing anticonvulsant ranges. Toxic levels of divalproex are potentially life threatening, although the risk is typically considered to be less when compared with lithium. Similar to lithium, divalproex comes in several formulations, including delayed release, capsule (sprinkle), syrup, and as an injection.

## CARBAMAZEPINE (TEGRETOL, EQUETRO)

Carbamazepine is a second-line agent for mania. Common side effects include nausea, vomiting, dizziness, drowsiness, and rash. Less common, but more serious, are liver damage, cardiac abnormalities, and decreases in red and white blood cell counts.

Carbamazepine is known to interact with multiple medications, requiring additional testing for drug levels and dosage adjustments. Routine blood-level monitoring is required for carbamazepine, utilizing anticonvulsant ranges and assessing blood cell count and thyroid function. Toxic levels of this anticonvulsant are potentially life threatening.

**LAMOTRIGINE (LAMICTAL)**

Lamotrigine is a first-line agent for bipolar depression in adolescents and adults. Common side effects include nausea, vomiting, constipation, ataxia, and skin rash. A serious dermatological side effect called Stevens-Johnson syndrome is associated with lamotrigine, especially when used in combination with divalproex. It is important to note that if lamotrigine treatment begins with very low and gradual dosing (a practice now mandated), rates of Stevens-Johnson syndrome are almost nil among adults and adolescents; however, it still occurs among preadolescent children. Benign rash, a common side effect of lamotrigine, may not be initially distinguishable from the more serious form. Patients and family members should be instructed to report any signs of rash to their physician. (See figures 3-C and 3-D.)

Although other anticonvulsants, including gabapentin (Neurontin) and topiramate (Topamax), are prescribed or mentioned in professional literature, these drugs do not have efficacy in treating either bipolar depression or mania. However, topiramate can be a useful adjunct to promote weight loss, and gabapentin can be useful to treat anxiety.

**OXCARBAZEPINE (TRILEPTAL)**

Oxcarbazepine is a third-line agent for bipolar disorder. It is an analogue (not metabolite) of carbamazepine and is believed to possess the same mechanism of action. Common side effects include sedation, dizziness, headache, ataxia, fatigue, nausea, dyspepsia, and double vision. Less common, but more serious, are hyponatremia (low sodium level) and rare activation of suicidal ideation. Although there is scant research on the use of oxcarbazepine in pediatric bipolar disorder, it is considered by some to likely be as effective as carbamazepine, and it has fewer side effects. Routine sodium level monitoring is recommended.

**TOPIRAMATE (TOPAMAX)**

Topiramate is a third-line agent for bipolar disorder. Common side effects include sedation, dizziness, anxiety, nausea, memory problems, confusion, decreased appetite, and weight loss. Less common, but more serious, are metabolic acidosis (excessive accumulation of acid in the body) and kidney stones.

The usefulness of topiramate in the treatment of bipolar disorder has less to do with controlling mania or depression and more to do with its side effects of decreased appetite and weight loss. The more effective medications for bipolar disorder (e.g., lithium, valproate) often lead to weight gain. Topiramate can be used adjunctively to counter this effect.

## ANTIPSYCHOTIC MEDICATIONS

All antipsychotic medications can treat mania (whether or not psychotic symptoms are present). In addition, two antipsychotics—quetiapine (Seroquel) and lurasidone (Latuda)—are FDA approved for treating bipolar depression. Antipsychotic medications have become popular choices in treating childhood mania. Geller et al. (2012) in the Treatment of Early Age Mania (TEAM Study) showed that monotherapy with either Depakote or lithium was not very effective (remission rates were 24 percent and 36 percent, respectively, hardly better than placebo response rates). The remission rate for risperidone (an antipsychotic, Risperdal) was 68 percent. See chapter 5 for a more detailed discussion of antipsychotics.

## *Guidelines for the Pharmacological Treatment of Bipolar Disorder*

Despite the fact that information is accumulating regarding treatment of early-onset bipolar disorder, only recently have experts begun issuing treatment guidelines (Kowatch et al., 2005). Most recommendations are based on case reports and open-label studies. There remains a critical need for definitive guidelines based on rigorous clinical drug trials that provide reliable information about safe and effective medication treatment for juvenile-onset bipolar disorder (Carlson et al., 2003). As is the case with adults, biological therapies for children include the use of mood stabilizers like lithium and anticonvulsants, antipsychotics, and electroconvulsive therapy (ECT). Treatment should be aimed at the stabilization of initial presenting target symptoms, full syndrome resolution, and relapse prevention.

The section below offers treatment guidelines for the phases (mania and depression), associated symptoms (agitation and psychosis), and comorbidities (ADHD and anxiety) of bipolar disorder.

**MANIA**

With acute manic episodes the first treatment consideration is to control severe agitation or hyperactivity. Standard treatments for this include benzodiazepines (minor tranquilizers, Ativan or Klonopin; note that the tranquilizer Xanax may aggravate mania) and/or antipsychotics. Minor tranquilizers can also lead to or worsen depression. The goal is to achieve behavioral control. In addition, treatment is started with mood stabilizers: lithium, divalproex, and atypical antipsychotics (e.g., quetiapine) are first-line agents. Therapy with a combination of mood stabilizers should be considered after careful evaluation; the majority of children with mania may ultimately require treatment with two or more mood stabilizers in combination to achieve a good outcome (Kowatch et al., 2000; Emslie & Mayes, 2001; Findling et al., 2003; Geller & DelBello, 2003). Similar to adults, polypharmacy (use of two or more medications to achieve a response or remission for a psychiatric condition) in children with bipolar disorder is more than likely the norm versus the exception.

**DEPRESSION**

There is general consensus that antidepressants are not effective in treating bipolar disorder and can actually worsen the condition (for example, by causing switches into mania and/or increasing the frequency of episodes). Currently there are six options for treating bipolar depression: (1) quetiapine (Seroquel); (2) lamotrigine (Lamictal) (can be used to treat adolescents, but caution is warranted in treating children owing to rare but dangerous side effects, such as severe rashes including Stevens-Johnson syndrome); (3) lithium, if given in doses large enough to achieve a blood level of at least 0.8 mEq/L; (4) olanzapine–fluoxetine combination (Symbyax); (5) lurasidone (Latuda); and (6) ECT for very severe, psychotic, and/or highly treatment-resistant cases.

## PSYCHOSIS AND AGITATION

Atypical antipsychotics are preferred.

## COMORBID ADHD AND BIPOLAR DISORDER

Initiate treatment with mood stabilizer(s). Once stability has been achieved, stimulants may be added gradually.

## COMORBID ANXIETY DISORDERS AND BIPOLAR DISORDER

The best medical treatments for anxiety disorders are antidepressants (e.g., SSRIs). However, as previously noted, these medications can destabilize bipolar disorder. Nonmedical approaches often provide good outcomes without the risk seen with antidepressants.

Treatments include cognitive-behavioral psychotherapy, exercise, and reduction or elimination of caffeine.

## *Manic Switching*

Current evidence provides conflicting information about the exact occurrence of manic switching and cycle acceleration with the use of antidepressants and stimulants. Experts have not determined precise risk factors in particular patient populations or disorders. Therefore, monitoring for mania or hypomania should be routine. Activation and disinhibition occur with antidepressants, and these side effects need to be differentiated from mania or hypomania.

| Drug | Typical Daily Dose | Side Effects |
|---|---|---|
| Lithium[1] | C[1]: 15–30 mg/kg in 3 or 4 divided doses<br>A[1]: 600–1,800 mg in 3 or 4 divided doses (or 2 divided doses for sustained-release products) | Sedation, thirst, gastrointestinal (GI) intolerance, tremor, weight gain in 30 to 40 percent of patients, hypothyroidism, headache, cognitive impairment, increased urination, acne, ECG changes, seizure<br><br>Dehydration can increase levels of lithium in the blood, which may be dangerous.<br><br>Children under 6 years old may experience more side effects. |
| Divalproex (Depakote)[2] | C and A: 10–60 mg/kg in 2 or 3 divided doses | Sedation, dizziness, drowsiness, blurred vision, lack of coordination, GI intolerance, rash, abnormal blood clotting, weight gain, hair loss, tremor, liver damage, pancreatitis, polycystic ovary disease |
| Carbamazepine (Tegretol) (Equetro)[2] | C: 10–20 mg/kg in 3 or 4 divided doses<br>A: 400–800 mg in 2 or 3 divided doses | Sedation, dizziness, drowsiness, blurred vision, lack of coordination, GI intolerance, rash, decrease in red and white blood cell counts, cardiac abnormalities |

| | | |
|---|---|---|
| Lamotrigine (Lamictal)[3] | C: contraindicated for use in children due to risk of Stevens-Johnson syndrome<br>A: complex dosing. Always starting at no more than 25 mg a day, with very gradual titration after week 2 | Dizziness, somnolence, headache, double vision, blurred vision, nausea, vomiting, and benign rash.<br>Rare: Stevens-Johnson syndrome |

C: prepubertal children; A: adolescents/adults.

1 Treats mania and bipolar depression.

2 Treats mania.

3 Treats bipolar depression.

Figure 3-C

# *Relapse Prevention*

Presently only a small body of literature describes the longitudinal course of bipolar disorder in children. In a 2-year follow-up study, Geller et al. (2002) reported that only 65 percent of patients reached full syndrome recovery, and 55 percent of those subjects ultimately relapsed. Biederman et al. (2003) reported similar results. Based on suggested remission types (Keck et al., 1998), Biederman et al. estimate that only 20 percent of bipolar youth had achieved functional remission or euthymia (normal, nondepressed mood) after 10 years. Boris Birmaher (2013) has studied the longitudinal trajectories for childhood-onset bipolar disorder. In a study lasting 8 years, he followed 438 bipolar children (average age of first episode was 9.3 years). Of those, 81.5 percent recovered from their initial episode, but this required prolonged treatment (an average of 2.5 years). During the 8-year timeframe, of those who recovered, 63 percent experienced recurrence (the average time to reoccurrence was 1.5 years). Birmaher's subjects represented different bipolar spectrum disorders: (1) bipolar I: 255 subjects, (2) bipolar II: 30, (3) bipolar NOS: 153. With long-term treatment (8 years), 24 percent achieved remission (euthymia), 19 percent were "much improved," 36 percent experienced mild to moderate recurring symptoms, and 20 percent remained ill. Factors associated with better outcomes included later onset of first episode, less family stress, higher socioeconomic status, less history of child abuse, less anxiety, and lower incidence of comorbid ADHD.

With adolescence and on into adulthood, long-term stability is only observed in less than 50 percent of those treated. This is owing to the significant side effects of bipolar drugs, negative stigma, and consequent poor medication adherence. Coletti, Leigh, Gallelli, & Kafantaris (2005) showed only a 34 percent medication adherence rate in youngsters treated for bipolar disorder. This strongly suggests that parents, who are responsible for administering medications, often have unspoken concerns about medical treatments. This in turn underscores the importance of appropriate education for parents regarding medications as well as the encouragement of ongoing, open communication about any and all concerns they have about their child's treatment. Such sobering statistics also reinforce the necessity of providing early and adequate treatment and ensuring compliance. Patient and family education should emphasize the necessity of long-term treatment.

Lifestyle management is a very important factor in achieving longterm recovery and should focus on the following:

- Maintain good sleeping habits (regular bedtimes and times for awakening; quiet evenings; limited exposure in the evening to light, like that which is emitted by computers and television) and avoid caffeine (including energy drinks).
- Get regular exercise (but not within 3 hours before retiring).
- At all costs, avoid substance abuse.
- Make wise decisions to not take on too much (e.g., college students should take a modest number of courses per semester).
- Actively address psychological issues and family stress with psychotherapy.
- Parents suffering from depression or other major psychological disorders should seek psychological treatment.

Additionally, the use of omega-3 fatty acids has been shown to afford benefits. For example, Melissa DelBello (2013) conducted a study of 56 depressed (unipolar) children. The double-blind, placebo-controlled study showed statistically significant benefits of omega-3 fatty acids compared with placebo. The dose of omega-3 was 1.2 grams (1,200mg) EPA and 0.6 grams (600mg) of DHA (docosahexaenoic acid). Note that omega-3 fatty acids derived from nut and seed oil have limited bioavailability in the brain (little across the blood–brain barrier), and EPA has a positive effect on mood regulation; DHA does not.

Bloch and Hannestad (2012) published a meta-analysis of omega-3 fatty acids to treat depression, in which positive effects were seen in doses of 1–2 grams of EPA. There is a general consensus that omega-3 fatty acids are less effective as an add-on treatment in bipolar disorder. Despite this, they are often recommended as a part of relapse prevention. (See chapter 9 for important safety information on over-the-counter products.)

As noted earlier, current discussion regarding early-onset bipolar disorder focuses less on its existence and more on diagnostic parameters and treatment options. Awareness of early-onset bipolar disorder is definitely on the increase. As noted earlier, some experts are questioning whether the pendulum has swung too far: is the diagnosis of childhood bipolar disorder being made too freely? Regardless, we aim to focus on the three themes common to both sides of the debate, detailed below.

First, it is generally accepted that bipolar disorder in juveniles is more severe than it is in adults. Early-onset bipolar disorder can have a negative impact on social functioning, school performance, and developmental progress. Second, underrecognition and inappropriate treatment leads to prolongation of intense suffering, may contribute to disease progression, and does not mitigate the suicide risk that may accompany adolescent bipolar disorder. Third, medications used to treat juvenile bipolar disorder are not innocuous and polypharmacy is common, underscoring the need for rational and careful use of these agents. All of these factors point to the importance of making an accurate diagnosis, selecting appropriate medications, and closely monitoring for therapeutic benefit and side effects.

| Drug | Interactions with Drugs Commonly Used in Pediatrics | Monitoring Parameters |
|---|---|---|
| Lithium | Increased lithium levels:<br>• Nonsteroidal anti-inflammatory agents<br>• Metronidazole (Flagyl)<br>Decreased lithium levels:<br>• Theophylline<br>Neurotoxicity*:<br>• Antipsychotics<br>• TCAs<br>• SSRIs<br>• Carbamazepine | Serum levels:<br>Acute mania: 0.8–1.5 mEq/L<br>Maintenance: 0.6–1.2 mEq/L<br>ECG, complete blood count (CBC), electrolytes, renal function tests, thyroid function, weight |
| Divalproex (Depakote [DVP]) | Erythromycin increases DVP levels.<br>DVP increases levels of TCAs.<br>DVP decreases levels of bupropion.<br>Risk of serious rash is increased when DVP and lamotrigine are taken together.<br>Variable effect on levels of other anticonvulsants when taken with DVP. | Serum levels: 50–150 mcg/ml<br>CBC, platelets, liver function, weight |

| | | |
|---|---|---|
| Carbamazepine (Tegretol [CBZ], Equatro) | Neurotoxicity*:<br>• Lithium<br>CBZ decreases levels/ effectiveness of:<br>• TCAs<br>• Antipsychotics<br>• Oral contraceptives<br>• Doxycycline | Serum levels: 8–12 mcg/ml CBC, ECG, liver function, weight |

* Although neurotoxicity can occur, it is infrequent and does not contraindicate combinations of lithium with the medications listed.

Figure 3-D

# CHAPTER 4

# Anxiety Disorders

Anxiety disorders are the most common psychiatric conditions in children, affecting 5 to 18 percent. These disorders result in significant academic and social impairment and often persist into adulthood. (It should be noted that anxiety disorders are frequently comorbid with bipolar disorder, depression, and ADHD.) In this chapter, we focus primarily on obsessive-compulsive disorder (OCD), since among the childhood anxiety disorders, OCD is one of the most well researched and one in which pharmacotherapy is a standard treatment strategy. Although medications can be useful for other anxiety disorders, they are often considered secondary interventions. These disorders will also be covered in the following pages with regard to pharmacological treatment.

# DIAGNOSTIC ISSUES

## *Obsessive-Compulsive Disorder*

The lifetime prevalence rate of OCD is 2.5 percent for adults and 1 to 2 percent for children and adolescents. In 25 percent of cases, OCD first emerges between the ages of 8 and 12. Other cases generally begin in late adolescence to young adulthood (mean age: 19.5 years). With childhood onset, the disorder is more common in boys than in girls (3:2 ratio). In adults, the gender ratio is 1:1. Onset is usually gradual, and the course of the disorder is chronic, with a waxing and waning pattern.

Symptoms of OCD include recurring obsessions (persistent and intrusive thoughts, ideas, or images that cause marked anxiety or distress) and compulsions (repetitive behaviors intended to reduce obsession-related anxiety). To meet criteria for a diagnosis of OCD, the obsessions and compulsions must be time-consuming (taking up more than one hour per day) and significantly disrupt normal routines, academic or occupational functioning, or relationships (criterion A). Obsessive thoughts are distinguishable from simple worry about everyday problems; children with OCD are not merely "worry warts." Frequently people with OCD avoid situations that involve obsessional content, such as public restrooms due to fear of contamination. They may feel driven to perform the compulsive behaviors, often according to rigid rules. Engaging in the compulsion relieves anxiety that builds up as a result of the obsession. Because there is intense shame, guilt, and secretiveness associated with OCD, diagnosis is difficult and often delayed. Many kids with OCD suffer in silence, and parents often feel helpless.

In adults, at some point during the course of the disorder, and with varying degrees of insight, they recognize the obsessions and compulsions to be excessive and unreasonable (criterion B). Note that criterion B is not a required diagnostic feature in children, as they may not possess sufficient cognitive awareness.

Common obsessions involve fears about disease and contamination, doubt, ordering, aggressive impulses, and religious and sexual imagery. Associated compulsions include handwashing, cleaning, checking, ordering, and mental acts such as silently counting or repeating words.

Childhood and adult OCD presentations are generally similar. In children, washing, checking, and ordering rituals and fear of catastrophe are particularly common. Compulsions without obsessions may occur in children, but generally do not occur in adolescents. Parents may become participants in their children's OCD rituals, especially when responding to reassurance-seeking behaviors, a form of verbal checking.

In a small subset of juvenile patients, OCD is associated with streptococcal infections such as scarlet fever or strep throat. The acronym PANDAS (pediatric autoimmune neuropsychiatric disorders associated with streptococcal infections) is used to identify this subgroup of the disorder. The proposed pathophysiology is a post-infection inflammatory process resulting in neuron damage in the basal ganglia. Characteristics include prepubertal onset and neurological abnormalities. Symptoms associated with PANDAS "come out of the blue" as opposed to developing or worsening over time. In fact, the acute aspect of PANDAS is one of its most distinguishing features. The primary focus of treatment is ridding the infection with antibiotics. (For a detailed review of this OCD subtype, see Snider & Swedo, 2004.)

## *Panic Disorder (With or Without Agoraphobia)*

The lifetime prevalence rate for panic disorder is 1 to 2 percent. Childhood onset is rare, with typical age of onset between late adolescence and mid-thirties. Panic disorder is characterized by recurrent, unexpected panic attacks and persistent worry and/or behavioral changes associated with the risk of additional attacks. Because panic disorder is so rare in children, emergence of panic attacks or panic-like symptoms may be an indication of severe psychosocial stressors (e.g., sexual abuse, domestic violence) or a medical issue (hyperthyroidism) warranting an appropriate evaluation. Panic disorder can manifest with or without agoraphobia. Agoraphobia is the fear of public places or situations that lead to feelings of being trapped and helpless. The child with agoraphobia may avoid going to birthday parties, movie theaters, playgrounds, or other areas where crowds gather.

## *Social Anxiety Disorder*

Lifetime prevalence rates range from 3 to 13 percent for social anxiety disorder. Prevalence reports may be upwardly affected by survey parameters, especially when fear of public speaking is included (the most common fear in American culture). The usual age of onset is in the mid-teens, often following a childhood history of social inhibition or shyness. Onset may be abrupt or insidious.

In social anxiety disorder, the sufferer experiences an intense fear of social situations, leading to anxiety and self-consciousness about being judged, criticized, or rejected. Social situations are very distressing, and the sufferer may avoid them entirely. Anticipatory anxiety and panic attacks are associated features. This anxiety disorder may result in failure to achieve, low self-esteem, and social isolation in children. The anxiety may manifest in crying, tantrums, and freezing in or shrinking from social situations. Diagnostically in children, the symptoms must occur in peer settings, not just with adults.

## *Specific Phobias*

Lifetime prevalence rates for specific phobias range from 5 to 12 percent. Initial symptoms usually occur in childhood, especially with the situational type, natural environment type, animal type, and blood-injection type.

A specific phobia is an enduring and unreasonable fear of a specific object or situation that usually poses little or no danger. Exposure causes immediate anxiety to the sufferer, who finds the object or situation very distressing and may avoid it entirely. Anticipatory anxiety and panic attacks are associated features. When children present with significant specific phobias, clinicians must always look carefully for underlying comorbidities, which are seen in the majority of cases (Walkup, 2004), and specific treatment considerations are required (Ollendick, Öst, Reuterskiöld, & Costa, 2010)

## *Generalized Anxiety Disorder*

The prevalence of generalized anxiety disorder (GAD) in children is between 2 and 6 percent and tends to occur more frequently in girls. GAD is characterized by excessive and exaggerated worry about everyday events. Anxiety and dread are so prominent as to interfere with daily functioning, including work, school, and social activities. Physical symptoms are common and include muscle tension, headaches, nausea, sweating, increased heart rate, insomnia, and exaggerated startle response. The cause of GAD is not fully known, but it is clear that severe psychosocial stress plays a role. Common examples of precipitating stressful events include the death of a loved one, divorce, physical and/or sexual abuse, and frequent geographical relocation.

## *Post-traumatic Stress Disorder*

The lifetime prevalence rate for post-traumatic stress disorder (PTSD) is 8.7 percent, with onset at any age, and usually within the first 3 months after a traumatic event. However, delayed onset may occur months or years later. PTSD develops when an event involving serious physical harm occurred, was threatened, was witnessed, or was learned about. It is important to note that beyond *DSM-5* criteria, other stressors may induce PTSD in certain individuals. How stressors are perceived (e.g., as being overwhelming or traumatic) is always in the eye of the beholder. Thus, PTSD may result from events such as abandonment, betrayal, severe humiliation, or bullying. Also, some people suffering from PTSD may be responding to states of helplessness or powerlessness, guilt, and shame. This is not uncommon in combat situations, where one's perceived inability to save, rescue, or protect others results in traumatic survivor's guilt or shame. This can also be seen in children who believe that they should be able to protect, for example, a parent or sibling who is the victim of domestic violence or sexual abuse. An area of controversy is that PTSD is a singular diagnosis in *DSM-5,* in that it *requires* specific stressors. All other diagnoses are simply syndromal, i.e., a set of symptoms without regard to etiology.

Typical reactions to traumatic events include shock, anger, anxiety, fear, and guilt. For people without PTSD, these reactions abate over time. For people suffering from PTSD, these symptoms continue, or increase, and interfere with functioning.

Technically, PTSD is no longer considered an anxiety disorder even though there is a strong anxiety component to the presentation. In the *DSM-5,* PTSD was included in a new category labeled "Trauma-and Stressor-Related Disorders." In part the move to the new category reflects the complexity of the disorder, which includes significant mood and behavioral symptoms.

PTSD symptomatology falls into four general clusters:

- Reliving: This includes flashbacks, disturbing dreams, and intrusive recollections. In children, repetitive play, event reenactment, or frightening dreams that do not directly refer to the traumatic event may be seen.
- Persistent avoidance and limited responsiveness: Efforts are made to avoid thoughts, activities, or places associated with the event. The sufferer may feel a sense of estrangement from others and have a restricted affective range. Children may have a sense of foreshortened future and a general withdrawal from normal life activities.

- Hyperarousal: Initial insomnia, hypervigilance, irritability, concentration problems, and exaggerated startle response may be seen. Children may experience stomachaches and headaches.
- Negative changes in thoughts, mood, and memory: Includes an inability to remember important aspects of the traumatic event; negative views about oneself, others, and the world; guilt and shame; depression; and isolation from others.

For a comprehensive review of assessment and treatment of PTSD in children, see *Treating Trauma and Traumatic Grief in Children and Adolescents, Second Edition* by Cohen, Mannarino, & Deblinger (2017).

## *Separation Anxiety Disorder*

Prevalence estimates for separation anxiety disorder are approximately 4 percent in children and young adolescents. (This disorder occurs only in childhood and adolescence.) When separated from home or primary attachment figures, children with this disorder demonstrate social withdrawal, apathy, and sadness. School avoidance often develops. Fear, anger, and attention-seeking behavior may also occur. Symptoms may wax and wane. The most notable presentation of this disorder is when a child has a difficult time separating from the parent when starting preschool, kindergarten, or first grade.

## *Adjustment Disorders*

Significant life stressors can provoke adjustment disorders that, by definition, are fairly short-term in duration. Also, such reactions, which often include anxiety symptoms and insomnia, typically cause suffering, but not serious impairment in functioning. These reactions often resolve over time without treatment, but if treatment is necessary, generally the approach of choice is psychotherapy. In some instances, very severe or tragic stressors (e.g., the sudden death of a parent) may result in intense anxiety. When this leads to insomnia, short-term use (a few nights) of a low dose of a tranquilizer (e.g., Ativan) or clonidine (e.g., Catapres or Kapvay) may be useful to help the child sleep. If symptoms are severe or persist, a referral to a mental health professional is in order.

## *Inhibited Temperament*

While not a *DSM-5* disorder, inhibited temperament is a genetically linked temperamental style (Biederman et al., 2001; Kagan, 1998; Schwartz, Snidman, & Kagan, 1999) that affects 10 to 15 percent of children and is characterized by the following behaviors or traits:

- Fear or withdrawal in unfamiliar situations
- Timidity and shyness
- Behavor inhibition
- Hypervigilance
- Autonomic arousal
- Association with a significant anxiety disorder later in life in approximately 30 percent of children with this temperament

# PSYCHOPHARMACOLOGY

## *Pharmacology of Obsessive-Compulsive Disorder*

SSRIs are first-line agents in the treatment of OCD. In addition, clomipramine (Anafranil), a TCA with serotonergic activity, is also highly effective in treating OCD. The relative side-effect profiles of an SSRI and Anafranil are often the determining factors in agent selection. (Anafranil has significant side effects such as sedation and weight gain.)

Response rates range from 50 to 75 percent, characterized by a gradual response pattern (Cook et al., 2001; Thomsen, Ebbesen, & Persson, 2001; Walkup, 2004).

| Time Course | Symptom Reduction |
|---|---|
| 6 to 10 weeks | 25 to 30 percent |
| 18 to 24 weeks | 40 to 50 percent |
| 52 weeks or more | 50 percent or more |

Figure 4-A

Generally, doses used to treat OCD are higher than those needed to treat depression. In figure 4-B, dosages are provided for medications used to treat pediatric OCD.

| Generic Name | Brand Name | Initial Dose | Daily Dose |
|---|---|---|---|
| Citalopram | Celexa | C/A: 10 mg | C/A: 10–60 mg |
| Clomipramine* | Anafranil | C/A: 25 mg daily | C/A: 200 mg or 3 mg/kg, whichever is lower |
| * FDA indication for children and adolescents | | | |
| Fluvoxamine* | Luvox | C/A: 25 mg at bedtime | C/A: 50–200 mg (higher doses divided) |
| * FDA indication for ages 8–17 years | | | |
| Fluoxetine* | Prozac | C: 10 mg daily<br>A: 10 mg daily | C: 10 mg<br>A (also higher-weight children): 20 mg |
| * FDA indication for ages 7–17 years. | | | |
| Sertraline* | Zoloft | C: 25 mg daily<br>A: 50 mg daily | C: 25–200 mg<br>A: 50–200 mg |

C: prepubertal children; A: adolescents/adults.

* FDA indication for ages 13–17 years.

** Before prescribing antidepressant medications to children or adolescents for OCD or related conditions, clinicians should consult FDA recommended dosing guidelines and practice-based guidelines such as *Stahl's Essential Psychopharmacology Prescriber's Guide: Children and Adolescents, First Edition* (2018).

Figure 4-B

# *Guidelines for the Pharmacological Treatment of OCD*

Pharmacotherapy for adult and pediatric OCD is solidly established, with similar response rates to medications for adult and pediatric OCD patients. Adequate dosages for extended periods of time are required. For adults, cognitive behavioral therapy (CBT) is a well-documented intervention, and response rates approach 90 percent. The most effective treatment for adult OCD combines medications with CBT.

The specific type of CBT employed in OCD includes exposure and response prevention. In this process the patient is gradually and systematically exposed to the anxiety-provoking stimuli but is not allowed to engage in the associated rituals. Initially, the experience is very difficult for the patient, but over time the drive to perform the rituals diminishes. Unfortunately, the technique is time-consuming and not readily available to all patients.

Until recently, the efficacy of CBT in childhood OCD relative to, or in combination with, medication was unclear. However, the Pediatric OCD Treatment Study (POTS), a 2004 multicenter NIMH-funded research endeavor, has provided clarity. Findings from this study suggest that treatment for pediatric OCD best begins with CBT alone, or CBT combined with an SSRI (Pediatric OCD Treatment Study Team, 2004). Further studies are needed to examine long-term outcomes and treatment guidelines.

In clinical practice, only a small percentage of children receive a recommended CBT protocol (March, Franklin, Nelson, & Foa, 2001). Most are placed on an SSRI as monotherapy. When adequate symptom response is not seen, the SSRI is sometimes augmented with clomipramine or an atypical antipsychotic. The latter is particularly true when OCD is accompanied by a tic disorder, which is a relatively common occurrence (Bloch, Landeros-Weisenberger, Kelmendi, et al., 2006).

# *Psychopharmacology of Post-traumatic Stress Disorder*

The treatment of choice for PTSD is psychotherapy. Empirically validated psychotherapies for PTSD generally include exposure (e.g., very gradually talking about or confronting the traumatic events). Exploring traumatic events can be risky because people suffering from PTSD can quickly become overwhelmed, experiencing a significant increase in symptoms and often dropping out of treatment. Four elements are necessary for successful exposure-based therapy:

1. Adequate ego strength and emotional resiliency (often assessed by a review of how well the child or teenager has typically coped with significant stress prior to the traumatic event)
2. A good support system (i.e., an understanding and supportive family)
3. A safe and solid therapeutic alliance with the therapist

4. Very gradual approaches to recalling and talking about traumatic experiences

Psychiatric medications may be used as an adjunct, focusing on three issues: (1) treating children who are very emotionally fragile or do not have an intact support network, (2) treating comorbidity (e.g., depression that often accompanies PTSD), and (3) enhancing the child's ability to better tolerate strong emotions. This can reduce symptoms to some degree and also may increase affect tolerance, better enabling the child to do exposure work.

Tranquilizers, although sometimes used for a very brief period of time in the immediate aftermath of a trauma, have not been shown to be effective for daily use beyond the first week or two after the trauma. And, in fact, longer-term use of tranquilizers can actually result in more severe symptoms over time. Two classes of psychiatric drugs that are helpful in improving emotional control (and are non-habit-forming) are SSRIs and alpha-2 adrenergic agonists (e.g., clonidine; see chapter 6 for more detailed discussion of these medications; also Connor, Grasso, Slivinsky, Pearson, & Banga, 2013). Even in the absence of depressive symptoms, SSRIs often reduce anxiety and enhance a child's ability to tolerate strong emotions. With SSRIs, it takes 3–4 weeks of treatment before the beginning of symptomatic improvement. Alpha-2 drugs may begin working in a few days (these medications must be started at low doses and gradually increased during the first week; dosing too rapidly can result in low blood pressure, dizziness, or fainting).

## *Psychopharmacology of Other Childhood Anxiety Disorders*

At this time the most convincing evidence to support medication treatment in other childhood anxiety disorders comes from the landmark Research Unit on Pediatric Psychopharmacology Anxiety study (Research Unit on Pediatric Psychopharmacology Anxiety Study

Group, 2001). In this multicenter, randomized, double-blind, placebo-controlled study conducted by a university-based research network, the safety and efficacy of psychiatric medications in pediatric patients were investigated. Anxiety symptom reduction was noted in 76 percent of the fluvoxamine (Luvox, an SSRI) subjects, with an effect size of 1.1 (one of the highest seen with any pediatric psychiatric disorder). The robust findings from this study strongly suggest a role for fluvoxamine in the short-term treatment of GAD, social anxiety, and childhood separation anxiety disorder (the authors also suggest that similar results are seen with other SSRIs, although fluvoxamine was the medication used in this study). Further studies are needed to replicate these very promising findings, and to amass a sufficient body of evidence from which to construct best-practice guidelines. Benzodiazepines also have a limited role in therapy, for short-term treatment when a child refuses to go to school or shows certain specific phobias, such as fear of dental or medical procedures.

Despite the dearth of evidence-based studies, clinicians often utilize SSRIs to treat a variety of childhood anxiety disorders, and all SSRIs appear to be effective in treating panic disorder, social anxiety, and GAD. When SSRIs are prescribed, initial dosages should be low, with a slow titration. As noted at the beginning of this chapter, for most childhood anxiety disorders, psychotherapy, including CBT, is the treatment of choice. However, psychopharmacological treatment of anxiety disorders in children is a rapidly emerging area of interest, and more findings will likely be published in the near future.

# CHAPTER 5

# Psychotic Disorders

Although psychotic disorders present relatively infrequently in childhood, they are usually a harbinger of lifelong illness. And late adolescence is a common time for first episodes of schizophrenia and bipolar disorder. (Bipolar disorder was discussed in detail in chapter 3.) It is rare to see schizophrenia in prepubertal children, because it more commonly presents in adolescence, and it has a lifetime prevalence rate of approximately 1 percent. Schizophrenia requires medical treatment not only for the acute psychotic episode, but also to prevent future episodes.

## DIAGNOSTIC ISSUES

Psychosis itself is not a diagnosis but a symptom. Historically the term has been defined, in *DSM-III-R,* as "gross impairment in reality testing and the creation of a new reality" (American

Psychiatric Association, 1987). Although a number of symptoms can be seen in the context of psychotic disorders, impaired reality testing is the central defining feature. Impaired reality testing may be seen in the form of bizarre behavior. However, it is most clearly observed in patients' verbal output and content of speech; psychotic patients reveal disorganized thought processes, false beliefs (delusions), and/or seriously impaired perceptions (hallucinations). Thus, depending on the person's age, psychotic symptoms may be more difficult to assess and detect in children, since they may be demonstrated only in their behavior, not in their verbalizations. You will note that the definition involves not only impairment of reality testing, which alone would simply lead to confusion, but also the "creation of a new reality," such as delusions ("I am being followed by a monster") or hallucinations ("I hear a voice telling me I am bad").

# TYPES OF CHILDHOOD PSYCHOTIC DISORDERS

Childhood psychotic disorders can be divided into three main groups: schizophrenia and related disorders, psychosis related to a mood disorder, and psychosis related to a medical disorder or substance abuse.

## *Schizophrenia*

Schizophrenia is a disorder that has been recognized since the time of Hippocrates. It can start during adolescence or, rarely, during childhood. A disorder previously called "childhood schizophrenia" included what is now considered autism (see chapter 7) and very rare forms of severe pediatric bipolar disorder.

The clinical picture of schizophrenia varies depending on the particular phase of the disorder. *DSM-5* divides the course of schizophrenia into three phases: prodromal, active, and residual.

During the prodromal phase, patients show deterioration in their level of functioning, or a failure to develop normally, without being actively psychotic. In this phase, the patient may show mostly "negative" symptoms (discussed below), such as a tendency toward isolation, blunted or flat affect, lack of initiative, and possibly a disruption of sleep patterns. Often the patient's school performance and personal hygiene deteriorate. This phase may last for months or years, making diagnosis difficult.

During the active phase, the patient shows psychotic symptoms with disorganized thinking, delusions, and hallucinations. This is often accompanied by anxiety and agitation.

In the residual phase, the patient continues to be impaired, but without florid psychotic symptoms. To warrant a diagnosis of schizophrenia, these three phases together must last at least 6 months. Schizophreniform disorder has the same criteria as schizophrenia, but its duration is less than 6 months.

For practical purposes, it is helpful to group schizophrenic symptoms into four categories, as outlined below. (Note that the characterological features are not psychotic symptoms by themselves but often accompany the core positive or negative symptoms.)

**POSITIVE SCHIZOPHRENIA SYMPTOMS**

- Hallucinations
- Delusions
- Agitation
- Floridly bizarre behavior

**NEGATIVE SCHIZOPHRENIA SYMPTOMS**

- Anhedonia
- Apathy
- Blunted affect
- Poverty of thought
- Feelings of emptiness
- Amotivational states

**DISORGANIZATION SCHIZOPHRENIA SYMPTOMS**

- Behavioral disorganization
- Distractibility
- Thought disorder

**CHARACTEROLOGICAL SCHIZOPHRENIA SYMPTOMS**

- Social isolation or alienation
- Marked feelings of inadequacy
- Poorly developed social skills

Other psychotic disorders include the following:

- Brief psychotic disorder: symptoms lasting less than 1 month, usually with an identifiable stressor
- Delusional disorder: persistent nonbizarre delusions
- Schizoaffective disorder: episodes of mania and/or depression in addition to the symptoms of schizophrenia
- Shared psychotic disorder: symptoms developing as a result of an intense relationship with someone who is already psychotic

## *Psychotic Mood Disorders*

Both depression and mania can present in children and adolescents with psychotic symptoms. Usually these are mood-congruent delusions or hallucinations. For example, depression may be accompanied by auditory hallucinations saying the person is bad or deserves to die, and mania may be accompanied by grandiose delusions. These are discussed in more detail in chapters 2 and 3.

## *Psychosis Associated with Substance Abuse or Medical Conditions*

Psychotic symptoms can be substance induced, or they can be related to a medical condition. Hallucinogens such as lysergic acid diethylamide (LSD), phencyclidine (PCP), and tetrahydrocannabinol (THC; see chapter 9 for a detailed discussion of marijuana/cannabis) can produce psychotic symptoms during intoxication, as can stimulants such as amphetamines, cocaine, or ecstasy. These substances can also lead to psychotic symptoms as a result of chronic use, particularly THC and amphetamines. Alcohol and sedative-hypnotics can produce psychotic symptoms during withdrawal.

# PSYCHOPHARMACOLOGY

There are two main types of antipsychotic medication: first-generation antipsychotics, also called *neuroleptics* or *FGAs: first-generation antipsychotics,* and the newer, atypical antipsychotics (SGAs: second-generation antipsychotics). These two classes of medications have significant differences with regard to side effects, which are described below. In general, the second-generation antipsychotics offer major benefits in the treatment of schizophrenia and psychosis related to a mood disorder. Psychosis related to a medical condition can be treated with a traditional antipsychotic. Other factors to consider include the following:

- If an antipsychotic medication has been used with success in the past (amelioration of symptoms and few side effects), generally the same medication is again prescribed.
- The patient's motor state is important to bear in mind. Typically, very agitated patients may be given a more sedating medication (such as Seroquel or Zyprexa), whereas markedly regressed or withdrawn patients will be given a less sedating drug (for example, Abilify or Geodon).
- The side-effect profile of the drug chosen must be considered in

relation to the individual patient's profile. For example, some of the atypical antipsychotics have a strong tendency to produce weight gain (discussed below) and should be avoided when treating a child who is obese or where there is a strong family history of diabetes.

## *Side Effects of Antipsychotic Medications*

Side effects from antipsychotic medications vary based on their molecular makeup and mechanism of action. High-potency antipsychotic medications (drugs that lead to a response at lower concentrations) generally result in more extrapyramidal or movement side effects and less anticholinergic, antihistaminic, and alpha-adrenergic effects (see below). Conversely, low-potency antipsychotics (drugs that require higher concentrations to achieve a response) typically result in fewer extrapyramidal side effects and more anticholinergic, antihistaminic, and alpha-adrenergic effects.

**EXTRAPYRAMIDAL**

In addition to producing a reduction in positive psychotic symptoms by blocking dopamine in the mesolimbic region, unfortunately, antipsychotics also produce extrapyramidal symptoms (EPS) by blocking dopamine in the basal ganglia. This is most true for the first-generation antipsychotics. The acute EPS are manifested as follows: (1) side effects resembling symptoms of Parkinson's disease, with slowed movements, decreased facial expression, resting tremor, and a shuffling gait; (2) dystonic symptoms, which involve sustained muscle spasms—usually of the neck or shoulder (such as torticollis)—and can be quite frightening and painful; and (3) akathisia, an intense feeling of restlessness. At times akathisia may be confused with psychotic agitation and lead to an increase in medication dosage—resulting in increased akathisia. Severe akathisia can be very uncomfortable and is associated with increased nonadherence and risk of suicide. Akathisia is most notable in those antipsychotic medications that tend to have less sedation as a side effect (e.g., Abilify, Geodon, Latuda). Antipsychotic medications, especially those that have high potency, can cause neuroleptic malignant syndrome (NMS), a potentially fatal neurological condition that is considered a severe form of EPS. Symptoms of NMS include high fever, tachycardia, muscle rigidity, and unstable blood pressure.

**ANTICHOLINERGIC**

Some antipsychotic medications block acetylcholine receptors and thereby affect the nervous system, leading to peripheral effects (dry membranes, particularly of the mouth and eyes; blurred vision, especially of nearby objects; constipation tachycardia; increased sweating; difficulty initiating urination; and sedation) and central effects (memory impairment, reduced concentration, and disorientation and confusion). Although the peripheral effects tend to be less severe, they are problematic for many patients and the primary reason antipsychotics are discontinued early.

## ANTIADRENERGIC

Some antipsychotic medications produce alpha-adrenergic blockade, which leads to orthostatic or postural hypotension. This means that when the child stands up, blood pressure drops significantly, leading to transient light-headedness, fainting, and potential injuries resulting from falls. Injury is most likely to happen during the middle of the night when the child goes to the bathroom or upon first waking in the morning. In order to minimize orthostatic hypotension and avoid injury, the child should sit on the side of the bed for a few minutes before standing.

## ANTIHISTAMINIC

The most common antihistaminic side effect associated with antipsychotics is sedation. Sedating medications taken during the day can lead to reduced focus and attention, sleepiness, and injury. If sedation is too great during the day, the medication can be taken at night. In fact, the sedating properties of antipsychotics can be exploited when insomnia is present. However, it is important to note that antipsychotics should generally not be used exclusively for insomnia because of the potential harsh side effects. Other common antihistaminic effects include increased appetite and restlessness.

## TARDIVE DYSKINESIA

All of the above-listed side effects appear within the first few hours or days of treatment or with increases in dose. In contrast, the tardive dyskinesias (disorders involving involuntary movements) appear late in the course of treatment or when the medication is reduced or discontinued. These movements usually lessen slowly over time, but they may persist for years even after the medication is discontinued. In some cases, they may be permanent. Patients should be routinely examined for tardive dyskinesia using the Abnormal Involuntary Movement Scale (AIMS; Munetz & Benjamin, 1988) or some other scale. The risk of tardive dyskinesia is significantly lower with the newer, atypical antipsychotics, although it is possible with higher-potency medications like Risperdal.

## METABOLIC

Recent concern about the SGAs has focused on their tendency to produce weight gain, type 2 diabetes, and an alteration of lipid metabolism. The elevation of serum lipids (triglycerides and low-density lipoprotein [LDL], or bad cholesterol) may lead to an increased risk of heart disease and stroke. The magnitude of this risk was discussed at a joint conference of the American Diabetes Association, the American Psychiatric Association, and the American Association of Clinical Endocrinologists (2004). The members of these organizations concluded that Clozaril and Zyprexa appear to have significant metabolic effects; Risperdal, Seroquel, and Invega appear to have moderate metabolic effects; and the other SGAs (Geodon, Abilify, Latuda, Fanapt, Saphris) appear to have minimal metabolic effects (although they have been less studied). They recommend that all patients on these medications should have their weight, blood sugar, and lipid levels assessed prior to starting a medication and monitored on a regular basis.

| ANTIPSYCHOTIC MEDICATIONS | | | | |
|---|---|---|---|---|
| **Generic Name** | **Brand Name** | **Initial Dose (mg)** | **Daily Dose (mg)[1]** | **Equivalence (mg)** |
| **Low Potency, First Generation** | | | | |
| Chlorpromazine | Thorazine | 10 | 150–375 | 100 |
| Thioridazine | Mellaril | 10 | 100–325 | 100 |
| **High Potency, First Generation** | | | | |
| Fluphenazine | Prolixin | 1 | 1.5–10 | 2 |
| Haloperidol | Haldol | 0.5 | 1–10 | 2 |
| Loxapine | Loxitane | 5 | 50–100 | 10 |
| Perphenazine | Trilafon | 2 | 6–22 | 10 |
| Pimozide | Orap | 0.25 | 1–5 | 1 |
| Thiothixene | Navane | 2 | 4–20 | 5 |
| Trifluoperazine | Stelazine | 1 | 2–15 | 5 |

| Generic Name | Brand Name | Initial Dose (mg) | Daily Dose (mg)[1] | Equivalence (mg) |
|---|---|---|---|---|
| **Second Generation** | | | | |
| Aripiprazole | Abilify | 5 | 10–20 | 10 |
| Asenapine | Saphris | 5 | 10–20 | 1–2 |
| Clozapine | Clozaril | 6.25 | 100–450 | 50 |
| Iloperidone | Fanapt | 2 | 12–24 | 10 |
| Lurasidone | Latuda | 20 | 40–80 | 10 |
| Olanzapine | Zyprexa | 1.25 | 5–15 | 2 |
| Paliperidone | Invega | 1 | 12 | 1–2 |
| Quetiapine | Seroquel | 12.5 | 100–550 | 50 |
| Risperidone | Risperdal | 0.25 | 0.5–4 | 1 |
| Ziprasidone | Geodon | 5 | 40–140 | 10 |

1 Doses appropriate for both children and adolescents.*

* Before prescribing antipsychotic medications to children or adolescents, clinicians should consult FDA-recommended dosing guidelines and practice-based guidelines such as *Stahl's Essential Psychopharmacology Prescriber's Guide: Children and Adolescents, First Edition* (2018).

Figure 5-A

| SIDE EFFECTS OF ANTIPSYCHOTIC MEDICATIONS | | | |
|---|---|---|---|
| **Medication** | **Sedation** | **Extrapyramidal** | **Anticholinergic** |
| **Low Potency, First Generation** | | | |
| Chlorpromazine | ++++ | ++ | ++++ |
| Thioridazine | ++++ | + | +++++ |
| **High Potency, First Generation** | | | |
| Fluphenazine | + | +++++ | ++ |
| Haloperidol | + | +++++ | + |
| Loxapine | + | +++ | ++ |
| Perphenazine | ++ | +++ | ++ |
| Pimozide | + | +++++ | + |
| Thiothixene | + | ++++ | ++ |
| Trifluoperazine | + | ++++ | ++ |
| **Second Generation** | | | |
| Aripiprazole | + | +/0 | 0 |
| Asenapine | + | + | + |
| Clozapine | ++++ | 0 | +++++ |
| Iloperidone | + | + | +/0 |
| Lurasidone | ++ | + | + |
| Olanzapine | ++ | +/0 | + |
| Paliperidone | + | + | +/0 |
| Quetiapine | ++ | +/0 | ++ |
| Risperidone | + | + | +/0 |
| Ziprasidone | + | + | + |
| Key: +++: substantial side effects; ++: moderate side effects; +: mild side effects; +/0: possible side effects; 0: none | | | |

Figure 5-B

# *Guidelines for the Pharmacological Treatment of Psychotic Disorders*

Because the child's psychotic behavior may be putting him or her in danger, paying attention to the child's safety in the initial evaluation is crucial. The clinician may determine that the patient needs hospitalization or other measures to ensure his or her safety. It is important to work with the family in this regard and to address any precipitating stressors. Antipsychotic medications should be considered at the first sign of psychotic symptoms, including disorganization of behavior. Often prompt initiation of treatment can help avoid the development of a more florid psychosis. Early intervention is important because psychosis is associated with increased suicide risk, and some evidence suggests that the longer a person is psychotic, the more difficult it becomes to treat the psychosis. The presence of delusional thinking, hallucinations, severe manic symptoms, or disorganized behavior suggests a need for antipsychotic medication. However, it is important to rule out substance use or medical conditions that may be responsible for the psychotic symptoms, prior to initiating antipsychotic medication treatment.

The first step in the initiation of treatment is to choose a medication, as discussed previously. The medication can then be started at a low dose, usually given at bedtime. (Note: One exception is Abilify, which is generally given in the morning.) The dose is then gradually increased until a good response is achieved or side effects become intolerable. If an effective dose is not tolerable, the clinician should try a new medication that would minimize the problematic side effects. For example, if the first medication produces severe EPS, a medication with low incidence of EPS should be tried. Generally, medication should be continued for at least 2 years after the first psychotic episode, but this will vary according to the specific symptoms, severity of the illness, and parental support.

Delays in treatment or discontinuing medications prematurely can result in more-severe psychotic symptoms and a disorder that quickly becomes harder to treat. When adolescents have their first psychotic episode, it is significantly disruptive to normal life, with time away from school and often a negative impact on the quality of friendships and family. Thus, a goal in treating a first episode is to reduce and eventually eliminate psychotic symptoms. However, beyond this, it is important to continue with medication treatment (typically for 2 years, as noted above). If there has been no recurrence of symptoms, then the antipsychotic may be gradually discontinued.

If the adolescent has a stable family situation and can be monitored closely, then the clinician can adopt a cautious, wait-and-see approach. Should any symptoms reemerge, it is essential to restart medication as soon as possible. Some teenagers with schizophrenia can recover from the initial episode and resume normal life (e.g., school, work, friendships). However, often when there is a second episode, it becomes significantly more difficult to reintegrate socially once symptoms have begun to subside. An alternative to medication discontinuation after the resolution of an initial episode is to continue with chronic medication treatment, but with a watchful eye toward side effects. Generally, after a second episode, most youngsters with schizophrenia must be treated with medications on an ongoing basis to prevent recurrent episodes and progressively worse psychosocial outcomes. In cases such as this, it is important to keep in mind that earlier treatment often leads to more chronic medication side effects such as tardive dyskinesia and metabolic dysregulation.

## Antipsychotic Medications and Children

From 2002 to 2009, prescriptions for antipsychotics (SGAs) increased by 65 percent, from 2.9 million to 4.8 million. Up to 90 percent of prescriptions were for "off-label use" (i.e., treating conditions for which the drugs did not have FDA approval; Jacobson, 2014, p.13). All antipsychotic medications are approved for treating schizophrenia; some are approved for treating bipolar disorder and for agitation and aggression in children who have neurodevelopmental disorders. They are often used to reduce severe aggression across a number of psychiatric and behavioral conditions (often with success).

However, these are not benign drugs. As mentioned above, many have significant side effects, especially metabolic effects (e.g., weight gain, increases in cholesterol and triglycerides, and increased risk of type 2 diabetes). Young people tend to be more susceptible to metabolic side effects, and there is already growing concern over escalating rates of childhood obesity. Clearly, psychotic symptoms cause great suffering and impairment and increase the risk of suicide, and they must be treated. However, it is important that prescribers carefully monitor for the emergence of side effects on an ongoing basis, use the lowest doses necessary, and periodically reevaluate to determine if continual treatment is warranted.

# CHAPTER 6

# Attention-Deficit/Hyperactivity Disorder

Attention-deficit/hyperactivity disorder (ADHD) affects approximately 5 to 7 percent of children. As teenagers mature neurologically, most with ADHD experience a no ticeable reduction in motoric restlessness or hyperactivity, but the core symptoms of ADHD (impulsivity, impaired attention, and lack of intrinsic motivation) continue through adolescence and on into adulthood. Most experts agree that about 40 percent of children with ADHD completely outgrow the disorder by early adulthood (likely due to the ongoing maturation of the prefrontal lobes, which may continue until the late twenties or early thirties). Of those with ADHD, 60 percent experience ongoing symptoms throughout life.

Medical treatments for ADHD are considered to be very effective, as we shall address below. Unfortunately, epidemiological studies have shown that approximately 5 percent of children meet criteria for ADHD, but only 13.6 percent of these have received treatment (Pliszka et al., 2000). Untreated ADHD results in considerable accumulated disability, and rates of co-occurring substance abuse, criminal behavior, anxiety, and depression are quite high Moreover, national health care costs associated with ADHD range between approximately $150 and $250 billion per year (Doshi et al., 2012).

## DIAGNOSTIC ISSUES

It is very important to emphasize the fact that most psychiatric disorders appearing in childhood present with some degree of motoric restlessness and inattention. Thus, these outwardly observable behaviors do not automatically lead to a diagnosis of ADHD. Figure 6-A lists those disorders that must be considered in any comprehensive evaluation of children with hyperactivity and inattention.

## DIFFERENTIAL DIAGNOSIS OF CHILDHOOD-ONSET PSYCHIATRIC DISORDERS PRESENTING WITH HYPERACTIVITY AND INATTENTION

- Diffuse brain damage (such as that commonly seen in fetal alcohol syndrome, following a head injury, and so on)
- Anxiety disorders
- Agitated depression
- Attachment disorders
- Situational stress/adjustment disorders
- Acute trauma
- Post-traumatic stress disorder
- Insomnia
- Bipolar mania or hypomania
- Prepsychotic conditions
- Impaired affect regulation associated with severe early abuse or neglect
- Substance use disorders
- Boredom (especially likely in bright children who are academically understimulated)

**Figure 6-A**

The diagnosis of ADHD is based largely on three sources of data: a detailed family history (since ADHD is considered to be a genetically transmitted disorder and thus often runs in families), a very careful history detailing the nature and onset of behavioral symptoms, and a description of current symptoms (especially as they vary across situations). It is also a diagnosis of exclusion; one must always first rule out those disorders listed in figure 6-A. Although psychological or neuropsychological testing can be helpful in diagnosing ADHD, it is not required. Some may argue that it is inappropriate to start a child on medication without formally assessing sustained attention and ruling out learning disorders and other psychiatric conditions. Although we agree that testing is important and can validate a clinician's diagnosis, the reality is that most children who are started on medication for ADHD do not receive formal testing. This makes the completion of a very thorough diagnostic interview and family review even more critical.

The most common presentation for ADHD is an early onset—often in infancy—of restlessness, unstable sleep patterns, and affective lability (especially excessive crying and difficulty being soothed). In most children, ADHD is identified when they enter preschool—where they experience their first sustained contact with other children and encounter social standards and expectations. Most experts agree that this *very early onset* of significant behavioral problems is characteristic of ADHD. However, emerging data suggest that some children destined to have bipolar disorder *may* show early-onset behaviors that are similar to ADHD (for example, prodromal symptoms of bipolar disorder; see chapter 3).

During childhood the following ADHD symptoms predominate: hyperactivity, impulsivity, impaired self-control, difficulty staying on task, and limited intrinsic motivation to stay focused, especially on mundane, non-exciting, or low-stimulus value tasks. Such symptoms are often highly context dependent; that is, they are most noticeable in situations where the child is required to remain still and quiet, such as in the classroom or church/synagogue, and they may not be as noticeable in an environment that is inherently exciting, novel, or stimulating, such as when playing sports or a video game.

With adolescence, as noted above, motoric hyperactivity is often reduced, but core symptoms remain. Disorganization, which may manifest in the form of messy lockers, notebooks, and bedrooms, is often pronounced in the ADHD adolescent, as are increasing problems adapting to societal and school-related demands for independent task performance and self-control. Additionally, rates of substance abuse are high, especially among untreated ADHD adolescents.

It is important to note that the so-called "inattentive" specifier of ADHD appears to be a totally unrelated neurological disorder. Children with this disorder do show impaired attention, but they are not hyperactive or impulsive. This fundamental difference is also underscored by the failure of stimulants to treat the inattentive subtype (except to a slight degree). Unfortunately, to date, there are no highly effective medical treatments for this inattentive subtype.

# PSYCHOPHARMACOLOGY

Three classes of medications have been shown through empirical methods to be effective in the treatment of ADHD: stimulants, certain antidepressants, and alpha-2 adrenergic agonists.

## *Stimulants*

Among the more than one hundred randomized controlled trials (RCTs) of stimulant treatment of ADHD, the results are very consistent: stimulant treatment of ADHD has a high degree of efficacy, with robust effect sizes ranging from 0.8 to 1.0 (Pliszka et al., 2000). Meta-analyses of several dozen RCTs of methlyphenidate revealed large effect sizes for children when rated by teachers and moderate effect sizes when rated by parents (Faraone et al., 2004).

The mechanism of action of stimulants is inhibition of dopamine reuptake (additionally, amphetamines promote increased release of dopamine from presynaptic vesicles). These drugs also increase the availability of norepinephrine in the frontal lobes. Figure 6-B lists currently available stimulants (with doses appropriate for both children and adolescents). There are different ways to categorize stimulants: either by the onset of action or by the duration of action. In general, most of these agents have a rapid onset of action, with symptom reduction occurring 30 to 60 minutes after ingestion, and a duration of action ranging from 4 to 12 hours (although most provide adequate symptom relief for only up to 6 hours). Depending on the formulation, dosing takes place two or three times daily, with some long-acting products requiring only oncedaily dosing. However, depending on the severity of symptoms and impact on functioning, long-acting medications may need to be dosed twice daily or combined with immediate-release formulations. It is most important to find the best possible dose and dosing schedule for a given patient.

There are three classes of stimulants: methylphenidate, amphetamine, and dextroamphetamine. (Note: Lisdexamfetamine is chemically related to dextroamphetamine.) Of children with ADHD, 38 percent appear to respond equally well to all stimulants; however, 62 percent have been shown to respond better to one specific stimulant than to others (Greenhill et al., 1996). What this means is that, although the stimulants are similar in their impact on the nervous system, differences do exist. Thus, if the results of a trial of one stimulant (such as methylphenidate) are less than optimal, then it is advisable to conduct a trial using another stimulant (such as dextroamphetamine). When systematic trials are conducted using each of the three classes of stimulants, good outcomes are seen in up to 90 percent of accurately diagnosed ADHD patients (Barkley, 2000). Overall, as noted by Falkowitz, Akbar, & Greenhill (2017), controlled studies on psychostimulants reveal that approximately 70 percent of patients have a significant response to psychostimulants versus around 13 percent for placebo. Arguably, no other class of psychotropic medications boasts this level of improvement.

## A FEW WORDS ABOUT STIMULANTS

Stimulants, in general, increase alertness, reduce drowsiness (ask any truck driver or college student), and help people to maintain focused attention. This is true for almost everyone and why it is not "diagnostic" when a child experiences these effects after taking a psychostimulant. The effects on psychologically normal functioning individuals are moderate and transient (usually lasting 3–6 hours). In children with the inattentive specifier, there may be only a slight improvement. In those with accurately diagnosed ADHD, the impact is robust.

| IMMEDIATE-RELEASE STIMULANTS* (duration of effect is 3 to 6 hours) | | |
|---|---|---|
| **Generic Name** | **Brand Name** | **Typical Daily Dose (mg)** |
| Methylphenidate | Ritalin<br>Metadate<br>Methylin | 10–60<br>10–60<br>10–60 |
| Dexmethylphenidate | Focalin | 5–20 |
| Dextroamphetamine | Dexedrine | 5–40 |
| Lisdexamfetamine | Vyvanse | 30–70 |
| Amphetamine | Amphetamine mixed salts (Adderall) | 5–40 |
| **SUSTAINED-RELEASE STIMULANTS* (duration of effect is 6 to 12 hours)** | | |
| **Generic Name** | **Brand Name** | **Typical Daily Dose (mg)** |
| Methylphenidate | Ritalin SR<br>Ritalin LA<br>Metadate ER<br>Metadate CD<br>Methylin ER<br>Concerta<br>Daytrana (patch)<br>Quillivant XR (liquid)<br>Aptensio XR<br>Contempla XR-ODT (orally disintegrating tablet) | 20–60<br>20–60<br>10–60<br>20–60<br>20–60<br>18–54<br>15–30<br>10–60<br>10–60<br>17.3–51.8 |
| Dexmethylphenidate | Focalin XR | 5–30 |
| Dextroamphetamine | Dexedrine spansules | 5–40 |
| Amphetamine | Adderall XR | 5–40 |

Figure 6-B

* Before prescribing psychostimulant medications to children or adolescents, clinicians should consult FDA-recommended dosing guidelines and practice-based guidelines such as *Stahl's Essential Psychopharmacology Prescriber's Guide: Children and Adolescents, First Edition* (2018).

Increasingly, stimulants are being used by those without psychiatric disorders as a sort of "performance enhancing" drug (i.e., to improve academic and occupational outcomes). However, in some individuals stimulants can provoke significant anxiety or precipitate panic attacks, and stimulants can increase psychotic symptoms in those with psychotic illnesses. As with all psychotropic medications (and all medications for that matter), there are risks.

Prescription stimulants are sometimes abused by those predisposed to substance abuse. However, it is important to note that children and adolescents with ADHD typically do not abuse these drugs. In fact, especially with teenagers, it is often difficult to get them to take the medications. Rather than getting a "buzz," most adolescents with ADHD report that stimulants make them feel somewhat "slowed down" (decreased spontaneity) and at times dysphoric. Some research suggests that the use of stimulants can reduce substance abuse in ADHD adolescents. It should be noted, however, that study results are mixed overall. Although most show significant protective effects (Biederman, Wilens, Mick, Spencer, & Faraone, 1999; Kuczenski & Segal, 2002; Mannuzza, Klein, & Moulton, 2003; Groenman et al., 2013), some show no difference in substance abuse rates when comparing treated and not treated ADHD teenagers (Sinclair, 2013). One major exception is that there are high rates of nicotine use among ADHD adolescents, whether treated or not.

In any case, the issue most important to be alert to is abuse by parents, siblings, and the child's friends (who may buy or steal the child's stimulants). Diversion of psychostimulants is not an uncommon occurrence. And because these meds are designated as a controlled substance by the Drug Enforcement Administration (DEA), this practice can lead to legal problems.

The prescription stimulants that have the lowest incidence of abuse are Concerta and Vyvanse. The antidepressants with ADHD efficacy (Strattera and Wellbutrin) and alpha-2 agonists (e.g., Kapvey, Intuniv, Catapres) are non-habit-forming and are generally not a concern with regard to abuse or diversion.

# *Guidelines for the Pharmacological Treatment of ADHD*

## STIMULANTS

Superior ADHD treatment outcomes for stimulants were demonstrated in a large-scale study (MTA Cooperative Group, 1999). Keys to successful treatment were shown to be the following: (1) start with low initial doses of stimulants; (2) carefully titrate the dose up to adequate levels; (3) dose three times a day initially (immediate release), then move to once or twice a day once an optimal dose is determined; (4) monitor for side effects; and (5) provide close follow-up. As noted above, stimulants produce noticeable symptomatic improvement 30 to 60 minutes after being ingested; thus, it is often possible to determine within a few days or a week which dose is most appropriate for any given child. Many children are treated for ADHD by their pediatricians, and close follow-up is rare, especially in managed-care settings. However, it is crucial, for optimal outcomes, to provide close supervision, especially during the first few weeks of treatment. If it is not possible for the clinician to see patients once a week, frequent telephone contact during the first few weeks of treatment can be very helpful. Additionally, it is important to monitor drug responses by using standardized rating scales that are completed each week by both the child's teacher and the parents (for example, the *Conners 3 Global Index for Parents and for Teachers,* Conners, 2008).

It is generally best to begin medication treatment during the weekend. Because the effects of stimulants generally last 4 to 6 hours, if treatment is started on a school day, the benefits of the medication may be noticed by teachers but will have worn off by the time the child returns home. Thus, the parents will not see the benefits and will be unable to provide an accurate assessment of the drug's effects. In fact, during the hour or two after the drug has been eliminated from the patient's body, there may actually be an increase in symptoms (this is referred to as "medication rebound effects"). As a result, the parents may witness only the problematic rebound behavior and decide to discontinue treatment.

There is general agreement among ADHD experts that stimulants should be used every day, not just on school days. ADHD, in addition to having a marked negative impact on academic performance, results in significant problems in social interaction. Children with ADHD are often loud, intrusive, and socially awkward ... in a word, *immature.* They may be the "class clown" but soon are seen as irritating and obnoxious and are rejected by other children. This social rejection is very painful for these youngsters. Appropriate, consistent stimulant treatment can significantly improve a child's social competency, peer acceptance, emotional interactions with family members, and self-esteem. Most children successfully treated with stimulants will require ongoing medication well into adolescence and possibly into adulthood. Stimulants are well tolerated and are considered to be the safest and have the mildest side effects of all psychiatric drugs. The most common side effects are initial insomnia (especially if administered after 4p.m. or if the child is taking sustained-release stimulants; see figure 6-B), reduced appetite, stomachaches, mild dysphoria, lethargy, and headaches. These side effects are usually easily managed (see figure 6-C).

Experts disagree regarding tics, ADHD, and stimulant treatment. ADHD and tics frequently co-occur (in both treated and untreated ADHD). In some instances, stimulants *may* exacerbate (but not cause) tics, even though in comparison studies the rate of tics seen in children treated with stimulants is not significantly different from placebo. Therefore, clinicians should tell parents that tic symptoms may increase but in most instances are not caused by the medication. Tics are commonly treated by the co-administration of alpha-2 adrenergic agonists.

Comorbid anxiety disorders are common in children with ADHD. Stimulants can, at times, exacerbate anxiety. However, a widely used and cited set of guidelines published by the Texas Department of Mental Health (Pliszka et al., 2000) recommends that, in cases of comorbid ADHD and anxiety, stimulants be used first. Often children's anxiety is associated with social and academic failure, and the anxiety subsides if the ADHD is successfully treated with stimulants. For patients whose anxiety increases significantly with a stimulant trial, it is a common practice to administer an SSRI along with the stimulant.

| STIMULANT SIDE EFFECTS AND SOLUTIONS | |
|---|---|
| **Side Effect** | **Solutions** |
| Initial insomnia | Try earlier dosing, or co-administer clonidine in the evening.<br>Do not administer sustained-release stimulants after 9 a.m. |
| Reduced appetite (Generally affects the patient only when the drug is active, and has not been associated with significant problems obtaining adequate nutrition; thus, is usually not treated.) | If necessary, switch to Focalin, which may result in less of this effect. |
| Stomachache | Give medications with food. |
| Mild dysphoria | Switch classes of stimulants, or add an antidepressant such as bupropion. |
| Lethargy, sedation, or impaired concentration (Generally indicates that the dose is too high.) | Reduce dose. |
| Headache | Reduce dose, or change stimulants. |

Figure 6-C

Many parents are understandably concerned about the use of stimulants since stimulants can be abused. It is important to openly discuss this issue with all parents and mention that treatment with stimulants may be associated with *reduced* rates of substance abuse, whereas failure to treat ADHD is associated with multiple personal failures (academic, interpersonal), family conflict, low self-esteem, depression, increased criminality, and *high* rates of substance abuse (often an adolescent's way of coping with depression and low self-esteem).

Parents have other concerns as well. During a period of 15 years, there were twenty-five cases of sudden death in children (in the United States and Canada) being treated with stimulants (Berger, Kugler, Thomas, & Friedberg, 2004; Vetter et al., 2008). Such deaths are considered rare. However, they understandably raised concerns and intense investigations. In all twenty-five children, upon autopsy there was evidence of preexisting, severe cardiac disease that had not yet been identified (that is, prior to death, none of these children exhibited noticeable signs or symptoms of heart disease). A number of studies have concluded from this that the role of stimulant use in these fatalities is unclear. Overall, stimulants have a track record of safety, with more than thirty years of use and millions of prescriptions (see the National Institute of Mental Health for more details: http://www.nimh.nih.gov).

It has become common practice to do cardiac screening (e.g., ECG) in children who present with any of the following: a family history of heart disease (i.e., heart disease in young or middle-aged adults, not elders), SIDS (sudden infant death syndrome), fetal alcohol or drug exposure, tachycardia (very rapid heart rate), dizziness, chest pain, or syncope (sudden, unexplained loss of consciousness). Absent these risk factors, generally, cardiac screening is unnecessary. However, considering that many parents have concerns about the health risks of psychostimulants and psychotropics in general, ordering a baseline ECG to reassure the parent and increase medication adherence seems reasonable.

## Medication Adherence in ADHD

One multisite study that looked at medication adherence in 254 children with ADHD showed only a 53 percent compliance rate (based on multiple, random salivary drug tests). Since parents administer these medications, such a low rate strongly suggests that those parents not following through with dosing instructions have concerns about the diagnosis and/or medication treatment. This underscores the need to proactively address any and all concerns that parents may have about medical treatment of ADHD (Pappadopulos et al., 2009).

One of the major drawbacks of stimulants is that they only work for a short period of time—if the medication is given in the morning, the positive effects wear off in the late afternoon. This presents a challenge, because ADHD symptoms can adversely affect patients in the late afternoon and evening, in the form of behavioral problems, family conflicts, or difficulty concentrating on homework. Also, when stimulants are taken after p.m., they commonly cause initial insomnia. Thus, co-administration of antidepressants or alpha-2 adrenergic agonists (see below) may be an option for targeting symptoms later in the day.

Mistaking other disorders for ADHD and treating these with stimulants can have highly adverse consequences (see figure 6-D).

| CONSEQUENCES OF MISDIAGNOSIS AND SUBSEQUENT STIMULANT TREATMENT | |
|---|---|
| **Correct Diagnosis** | **Consequences** |
| Anxiety disorder | Increased anxiety |
| Agitated depression | Increased agitation |
| Preschizophrenia | Psychosis |
| Bipolar disorder | Increased manic symptoms<br>*Possible* cycle acceleration |
| Situational stress | Failure to address psychological issues |
| Depression | Increased apathy and dysphoria |
| Insomnia | Increased difficulty initiating or maintaining sleep |

Figure 6-D

Bipolar disorder and ADHD are often co-occurring. Stimulants prescribed (without mood stabilizers) to bipolar youngsters can sometimes cause significant problems (e.g., intensifying manic symptoms or contributing to rapid cycling). However, it is generally accepted that once a child with bipolar disorder is well controlled on mood stabilizers or antipsychotics, stimulants may be added that improve ADHD symptoms and do not seem to aggravate bipolar symptoms.

## ALPHA-2 ADRENERGIC AGONISTS

Clonidine (Catapres, Kapvay) and guanfacine (Tenex, Intuniv) may be used to treat core ADHD symptoms (see figure 6-E); however, they are more effective in reducing irritability, aggression, and impulsivity and promoting sedation (to treat initial insomnia). Alpha-2 agonists are also the treatment of choice for comorbid tics.

ALPHA-2 ADRENERGIC AGONISTS

| Generic | Brand | Typical Dose[1] |
|---|---|---|
| Clonidine | Catapres<br>Kapvay | 0.15–0.4 mg[2]<br>0.15–0.4 mg |
| Guanfacine | Tenex<br>Intuniv | 0.25–3.0 mg[3]<br>0.25–3.0 mg |

1 Doses appropriate for children and adolescents

2 Three to four times a day

3 Two to three times a day

Figure 6-E

Combined use of alpha-2 agonists and stimulants is a common practice, both for treating ADHD alone and comorbid ADHD and tics (Walkup, 2004). Although four cases of death in children taking clonidine in conjunction with a stimulant have been reported, the FDA conducted an investigation and failed to find any significant cause for concern over the co-administration of these drugs. The deaths occurred in children with very complicated medical problems, and the FDA concluded that the drugs were not a causal factor in the deaths.

## ANTIDEPRESSANTS

Of children with ADHD, 20 percent will experience co-occurring depression. Antidepressants certainly may be helpful in reducing mood symptoms. However, certain classes of antidepressants have also been shown to have positive effects on core ADHD symptoms. Not all antidepressants should be used to treat ADHD—only those that increase the availability of dopamine or norepinephrine. Thus, SSRIs, although often a good adjunct for treating anxiety or depression, are not effective in treating core ADHD symptoms. In fact, as mentioned in chapter 2, a later-onset side effect of SSRIs can be disinhibition. When this occurs in patients being treated for ADHD, it can result in an increase in impulsivity and occasionally aggression. Therefore, while SSRIs are not contraindicated in the treatment of comorbid anxiety or depression, the clinician must be watchful for this possible complication. Antidepressants that have evidence of efficacy in treating ADHD are listed in figure 6-F. (Note that tricyclic antidepressants have been found to be effective in treating ADHD; however, due to significant side effects and toxicity, these are not generally drugs of choice. In some treatment-resistant cases, nortriptyline can be used as an alternative.)

| ANTIDEPRESSANTS USED TO TREAT ADHD | | |
|---|---|---|
| **Generic Name** | **Brand Name** | **Typical Daily Dose** |
| Bupropion | Wellbutrin SR/LA | $C_1$: 100–150 mg<br>$A_1$: 150–300 mg |
| Atomoxetine | Strattera | 1.2–1.8 mg/kg (same for children and adolescents) |
| C: prepubertal children; A: adolescents/adults. | | |
| Figure 6-F | | |

Treatment outcomes with antidepressants for ADHD symptoms are not as robust as those seen with stimulants; however, antidepressants afford several advantages:

- Once-a-day dosing
- No need for triplicate prescription
- No addiction potential
- Effects (generally seen within 5 to 40 days after initiating treatment) typically last 24 hours and thus cover evening hours
- Can be used to treat comorbid depression

Antidepressants generally require a low starting dose and a gradual increase over the first 3 weeks of treatment. Although some positive effects can be seen in the first 1 to 3 weeks, achieving the full effect may require 3 months of ongoing treatment.

## COMBINED BEHAVIORAL TREATMENT AND PSYCHOPHARMACOLOGY

The MTA Study (Multimodal Treatment Study of Children with ADHD) demonstrated that medication treatment alone was as effective as behavioral treatment and that the combination of both treatment modalities provided only modest benefits beyond the use of each treatment separately (MTA Cooperative

Group, 1999). However, in most cases the ideal treatment is to use both medication and psychological approaches to manage core ADHD symptoms. And certainly psychotherapy (family and/or individual) can be very helpful in treating comorbid anxiety or depression.

# CHAPTER 7

# Autism Spectrum Disorder

Autism spectrum disorder (ASD) represents a class of neurodevelopmental disorders. These include classic autism and Asperger's syndrome (note that in this discussion we have also included Rett's disorder and childhood disintegrative disorder; both are rare neurodevelopmental disorders, not considered to be related to autism). The prevalence rate of ASD in the United States is approximately 1 percent (American Psychiatric Association, 2013, p.55). These disorders manifest in various degrees of dysfunction in four main areas: social interaction, communication, emotional regulation, and repetitive behaviors. Boys are three to four times more likely than girls to have autism. ASD was originally thought to be more common in upper socioeconomic classes, but more recent studies suggest that this was due to referral bias and greater access to care for more affluent families. Currently, these disorders are under intense investigation due to their prevalence and the lack of effective specific treatments. It is hoped that a better understanding of them will lead to a clearer picture of the relationship between the brain and behavior.

# DIAGNOSTIC ISSUES

## *Autism*

Autism (a common term used to refer to both autism and autistic disorder) was originally described in a series of eleven case histories by Leo Kanner (1943), who gave it the name *early infantile autism* and identified two main features: autistic aloneness and obsessive insistence on sameness. The abbreviated term "infantile autism" made its way into the *DSM-III* in 1980 (American Psychiatric Association, 1980). Since then, many revisions have been made to the diagnostic criteria. Recent revisions in diagnostic criteria require impairment in the areas of social interaction, communication, and stereotyped behavior, as listed below:

1. Significant impairment in social interaction, such as the following:
    - Impairment in the use of nonverbal behaviors such as facial expression
    - Failure to develop peer relationships appropriate to age
    - A lack of spontaneous seeking to share interests with others
2. Significant impairments in communication, as shown by at least one of the following:
    - Delayed or absent development of spoken language
    - In individuals with adequate speech, impaired ability to converse with others
    - Use of language in stereotyped or idiosyncratic ways
    - Lack of make-believe play or imitative play appropriate to age
3. Stereotyped patterns of interests and activities, as shown by at least one of the following:
    - Intense preoccupation with one or more stereotyped and restricted patterns of interest

- Rigid adherence to nonfunctional routines or rituals
- Stereotyped and repetitive motor mannerisms
- Intense preoccupation with parts of objects

A number of rating scales are used to screen for and diagnose autistic disorder: the Autism Behavior Checklist (ABC), Autism Diagnostic Observation Schedule (ADOS), Autism Screening Questionnaire (ASQ), Autism Spectrum Screening Questionnaire (ASSQ), Checklist for Autism in Toddlers (CHAT), Childhood Autism Rating Scale (CARS), and Autism Diagnostic Interview (ADI).

Autism needs to be differentiated from Asperger's syndrome, Rett's disorder, childhood disintegrative disorder, and other developmental disorders such as severe intellectual disabilities and developmental language disorders. The distinguishing features will be discussed below. In addition, autism is often associated with a variety disorders. It appears to be most closely related to anxiety disorders, as anxiety, fears, sleep problems, and obsessive-compulsive symptoms are common. Also, attentional problems, hyperactivity, self-injurious behavior, mood symptoms, and tics are fairly common.

## *Asperger's Syndrome*

Asperger's syndrome is often considered a mild form of autism, first described by Hans Asperger in 1944 (Asperger, 1991). In Asperger's, as in autism, there is impairment in social relationships and repetitive and stereotyped patterns of behavior, but minimal delay in language development. People with Asperger's are interested in social relationships but are socially clumsy and insensitive. Distinguishing between high-functioning autism and Asperger's can be difficult. The following are diagnostic features of Asperger's disorder:

1. Qualitative impairment in social interaction, as manifested by at least two of the following:
   - Impairment in the use of nonverbal behaviors such as facial expression

- Failure to develop peer relationships appropriate to age
- Lack of spontaneous seeking to share interests with other people
- Lack of social or emotional reciprocity

2. Stereotyped patterns of interests and activities, as shown by at least one of the following:
   - Intense preoccupation with one or more stereotyped and restricted patterns of interest
   - Rigid adherence to nonfunctional routines or rituals
   - Stereotyped and repetitive motor mannerisms
3. The disturbance causes clinically significant impairment in social, occupational, or other important areas of functioning.
4. No clinically significant delay in language is seen.

## *Rett's Disorder*

Rett's disorder was first described by Andreas Rett in 1966 (Rett, 1977). A condition characterized by its developmental course and development of neurological and behavioral symptoms, it has been linked to mutations in the gene encoding X-linked methyl-CpG-binding protein 2 (MECP2) and is seen almost exclusively in females. There are several types of mutations of the *MECP2* gene, but the relationship between type of mutation and clinical presentation is unclear at this time. Those with the disorder do not show any symptoms until after the age of 5 months. Subsequently, children with Rett's develop stereotyped hand movements, impaired social interaction, lack of coordination, and impaired language ability. Following are the diagnostic criteria:

1. All of the following:
    - Apparently normal prenatal and perinatal development
    - Apparently normal psychomotor development through the first 5 months after birth
    - Normal head circumference at birth
2. The following appear after the period of normal development:
    - Reduced head growth between 5 and 48 months

- Loss of previously acquired hand skills, between ages 5 and 30 months and the development of stereotyped hand movements
- Early loss of social engagement (although social interaction may develop later)
- Development of poorly coordinated gait or trunk movements
- Severely impaired language development

Rett's disorder is associated with abnormal sleep patterns, cardiac and respiratory abnormalities, epilepsy, a variety of behavioral and emotional problems, and increased mortality (Kerr, Armstrong, Prescott, Doyle, & Kearney, 1997).

## *Childhood Disintegrative Disorder*

This disorder was first described by Theodore Heller (1908) and has been referred to as "Heller's syndrome." It now appears in the *DSM-5* under the category "Other Specified Neurodevelopmental Disorders." Children with this disorder develop normally until at least age 3 or 4 years and then, sometimes following encephalitis, deteriorate over a period of weeks or months. They show significant loss of language ability, social skills, intellectual functioning, and bowel or bladder control and develop repetitive movements and mannerisms. After a period of deterioration, they stabilize and do not show further loss of function. The disorder is seen mainly in males, and is rare. Currently there are no well-established pharmacological treatments for childhood disintegrative disorder.

## *Reactive Attachment Disorder*

Reactive attachment disorder of infancy or childhood is not considered to be a neurodevelopmental disorder. It is presumed that this syndrome can develop as a response to severe early neglect or abuse. There is a pattern of withdrawal from the caregiver; little expression of positive feelings; and unexplained, intense emotional reactions such as irritability, sadness, or fearfulness in the absence of provoking stressors. Additionally, these children rarely if ever seek protection or comfort from caregivers (American Psychiatric Association, 2013). Although it is listed in the *DSM-5* category "Trauma and Stressor-Related Disorders," rather than neurodevelopmental disorders, this does not imply that there is no underlying neurobiological aspect to the disorder. It has been clearly established that severe early neglect or abuse can result in not only behavioral and social impairment, but also persistent neurological dysfunction. Currently there are no well-established pharmacological treatments for reactive attachment disorder.

# PSYCHOPHARMACOLOGY

## *Guidelines for the Pharmacological Treatment of Pervasive*

# *Neurodevelopmental Disorders*

The treatment of neurodevelopmental disorders involves a team approach. It is important that parents and other caregivers, educators, speech therapists, occupational therapists, psychologists, pediatricians, and psychiatrists all work together closely. The main part of the habilitation process involves behavioral and educational interventions. Medication is used mainly to control symptoms sufficiently to allow the interventions to progress as opposed to "correcting" an underlying neurobiological cause.

There is no effective medication treatment specific to any of the ASDs. Certain types of medications have been shown to sometimes be beneficial in the treatment or control of associated symptoms of the pervasive neurodevelopmental disorders (PNDs). These are discussed below.

## SEROTONERGIC MEDICATIONS

A type of medication commonly used in the treatment of the PNDs is the group of serotonergic antidepressants, including the SSRIs. These medications are often helpful in reducing aggression, agitation, ritualistic behavior, mood symptoms, and anxiety. Medications within this class that have the most research supporting their use include fluoxetine, fluvoxamine, and sertraline. It's generally believed that all SSRIs are likely equally efficacious in the alleviation of PND symptoms. The tricyclic antidepressant clomipramine, a highly serotonergic medication approved for the treatment of obsessive-compulsive disorder in children, has also been shown to be useful in PND-associated aggression, repetitive behavior, and social engagement (Brodkin et al., 1997). SSRIs are discussed in detail in chapter 2, and clomipramine is discussed in chapter 4.

**ANTIPSYCHOTICS**

Antipsychotic medications are also often used in the treatment of PNDs. They can be helpful in reducing aggression and agitation and improving social relatedness. Because of the risk of extrapyramidal symptoms and tardive dyskinesia with long-term use of the earlier antipsychotics, the second-generation antipsychotics are preferred. Risperidone and aripiprazole have the most available data supporting their use. Risperidone has been shown to improve social relatedness, repetitive thoughts, and other PND-related behavior (Purdon, Wilson, Labelle, & Jones, 1994; McDougle et al., 1998; Kent et al., 2013). Aripiprazole is FDA approved for the treatment of autism-related irritability in children ages 6 to 17 and is supported by multiple clinical trials (Palumbo, Keary, & McDougle, 2017). Although the results have been encouraging, some evidence indicates that children may be more sensitive to extrapyramidal and cardiac side effects and metabolic effects such as weight gain and increased blood sugar levels. These medications are discussed in detail in chapter 5.

## BETA-BLOCKERS AND ALPHA-2 AGONISTS

Beta-blockers are considered antihypertensives and are effective in reducing blood pressure because they block one type of norepinephrine receptor. They have been reported to reduce aggression, impulsivity, anxiety, and self-injurious behavior in a variety of clinical presentations. However, research on the use of this class of medication in children with PNDs is sparse. Similarly, clonidine and guanfacine, medications that also reduce blood pressure, have been shown to have a calming effect. Extended-release versions of these medications are approved to treat ADHD in children between the ages of 6 and 17 and have been shown to reduce hyperactivity in autism and related conditions.

## MOOD STABILIZERS

There may be some role for lithium and anticonvulsants (Depakote and Tegretol) in the control of agitation, aggression, and self-harm (e.g., head-banging or biting oneself). However, these medications are generally not first-line interventions due to side effects, laboratory monitoring, and potential toxicity. These medications are discussed in detail in chapter 3.

## STIMULANTS

Psychostimulants are sometimes helpful in the treatment of attentional problems in children with a PND. Because of the risk of increased agitation and excitability, they must be used with caution, and usually in low doses. Stimulants should be used only when the child has a generalized problem with distractibility, and not when the distraction is due to preoccupation with some type of ritualistic behavior. These medications are discussed in detail in chapter 6.

## OPIOID ANTAGONISTS

Some reports have indicated that naltrexone, an opiate blocker, may be effective in reducing restlessness and improving focus (Kolmen, Feldman, Handen, & Janosky, 1995), but controlled studies have not shown consistent benefit (Campbell et al., 1993).

## OXYTOCIN

Oxytocin is a hormone that has been found to influence social bonding. There are a number of randomized clinical trials using oxytocin (often administered via nasal infusion [nasal spray]) that show some promise in improving social recognition and learning (for example, enhancing the ability of individuals with autism to learn to recognize emotional facial expressions) and other PND-related behaviors; however, the data are mixed (Preti et al., 2014). Note that nasal spray for oxytocin is FDA approved for use in promoting labor and to facilitate the release of milk in breastfeeding women; it is not approved for the treatment of ASD. But again, the nasal spray formulation has shown some promise in recent studies evaluating the efficacy of oxytocin in treating autism. (Early studies used injectable oxytocin, but nasal infusion is easier to administer.)

## MISCELLANEOUS AGENTS

The intense interest in autism and related disorders has stimulated much research into potentially effective treatments. Currently the main approach to treatment is to use medications appropriate to the associated conditions, such as an SSRI when there are prominent obsessive-compulsive symptoms. The following treatments have been proposed, but without sufficient evidence to support their efficacy:

- D-cycloserine, a broad-spectrum antibiotic used to treat tuberculosis
- Secretin, a gastrointestinal hormone
- Digestive enzymes
- Levetiracetam, an anticonvulsant, reported to reduce hyperactivity, impulsivity, mood instability, and aggression
- Donepezil, a cholinesterase inhibitor used in the treatment of Alzheimer's disease, reported to reduce irritability and hyperactivity
- Thiamine tetrahydrofurfuryl disulfide (TTFD), proposed due to its ability to counteract the effect of heavy metals, such as mercury in thimerosal
- Carnosine, a dipeptide with neurological activity
- Lofexidine, an alpha-adrenergic receptor partial agonist similar to clonidine, shown to have some benefit in reducing hyperactivity
- Tianeptine, to reduce irritability in children with autistic disorder

# *Initiating Treatment*

The initial choice of medication should be based on the type of symptoms that are interfering most with the child's habilitation progress, side-effect profile, and wishes of the child and parents or guardians. Once chosen, the medication should be started at a low dose and monitored closely for effects, both positive and negative.

# CHAPTER 8

# Sleep Disorders

According to Shakespeare, sleep is the "bath and balm of hurt minds." Sleep disturbances can occur with almost all psychiatric conditions (e.g., situational stress/adjustment disorders, anxiety disorders, PTSD, depression, and bipolar disorder) as well as with primary sleep disorders. Poor or inadequate sleep is oft en not identified in many children and teens seeking psychological or psychiatric treatment, and is a common reason for less than adequate outcomes. One problem is that many parents simply do not know how well their child sleeps. Going to bed on time is one thing, but various forms of insomnia and other sleep problems may never be mentioned by youngsters, so their parents may not know that a problem exists.

# DIAGNOSTIC ISSUES

## *Insomnia*

It has been estimated that up to 25 percent of children and adolescents experience some form of sleep disturbance, with approximately one out of five children between the ages of 5 and 12 experiencing insomnia specifically (Calhoun et al., 2014). Insomnia is generally characterized as manifesting in one of three ways.

The first is *initial insomnia,* or trouble falling asleep. Initial insomnia is a common reaction to situational stress and is seen in most types of anxiety disorders. The child or adolescent experiencing this type of sleep difficulty may ruminate about school, family, social relationships, or anything else that may be troubling them. Most commonly this is done while lying in bed. Even though the child may be sleepy, the drive to engage in ruminative behavior is often stronger than the desire to sleep. Moreover, over time, lying in bed while worrying or thinking about things will become a learned behavior (habit) leading to significant reductions in quantity of sleep.

*Middle insomnia* (waking up numerous times during the night) can also be associated with anxiety, but is most often related to depression. The child with middle insomnia may have little difficulty falling asleep, but may wake up several times throughout the night. Generally the child is able to fall back to sleep, but deficits in both quantity and quality of sleep leave the child feeling tired and run down the following day. Nightmares associated with post-traumatic stress disorder can also contribute to frequent nighttime awakenings.

Early morning awakening, often referred to as *terminal insomnia,* is frequently seen in children suffering from depression. The child may have little problem falling asleep and is able to sleep for several hours, but wakes hours before his or her scheduled wake time. Unfortunately, going back to sleep is difficult if not impossible.

It is important to note that decreased need for sleep is a hallmark of mania and hypomania. Unlike a child with initial, middle, and terminal insomnia, the child suffering from mania or hypomania does not feel the need to sleep.

## *Nightmare Disorder*

Most everyone has a nightmare at some point, and this is generally of little clinical significance. However, a small but significant percentage of children will have nightmares on a regular basis. The prevalence of having at least one nightmare a week has been estimated to be as high as 5 percent (Li et al., 2011). Up to 4 percent of mothers indicate their preschool children have nightmares "often" or "always" (Simard, Nielsen, Tremblay, Boivin, & Montplaisir, 2008).

Nightmares in children are often reported as dysphoric and threatening in nature. Nightmares are generally vivid, and upon wakening, the child is able to recall much of the narrative of the dream. Although nightmares are often associated with acute and chronic physical and psychological trauma, this is not always the case. Nightmares can arise from daily life stress or occur in the absence of any identifiable stressor.

Nightmares cause significant disruption in a child's daily life in two primary ways. First, nightmares result in fragmented and disrupted sleep. Moreover, after having a nightmare, the child may be so upset and fearful that he or she isn't able to fall back to sleep. This leaves the child feeling tired and run down the following day. Consequently, schoolwork, social relationships, and family responsibilities may suffer. And second, the dysphoric mood associated with a nightmare often follows the child into the day, leaving him or her feeling depressed, anxious, and/or irritable.

## *Obstructive Sleep Apnea*

Obstructive sleep apnea (OSA) is a sleep disorder characterized by a partial or complete cessation of breathing while sleeping. The prevalence of pediatric OSA is approximately 3 percent and is often seen in children who are significantly overweight (excessive fat around the neck restricts breathing while lying down) or who have enlarged adenoids and tonsils.

Unlike adults with OSA, daytime fatigue and sleepiness are not the most common complaints. Behavioral disturbances are generally seen in children with OSA as well as poor performance at school, irritability, and impairments in attention and concentration. In fact, the manifestation of OSA in children is different depending on the age of the child.

The following are some key diagnostic features of OSA by age range (Chang & Chae, 2010):

**Infant**

- Disturbed sleep with crying upon awakening
- Snoring or loud breathing
- Sweating while asleep
- Developmental delays
- Reduced sucking reflex

**Toddler**

- Snoring or loud breathing
- Restless sleep
- Strange sleeping positions
- Breathing through the mouth

- Night terrors
- Developmental delays

**Preschool children**

- Heavy, loud snoring
- Breathing from the mouth
- Excessive dry mouth upon awakening
- Bedwetting
- Poor daytime attention

**School-aged children**

- Heavy, loud snoring
- Bruxism (teeth grinding)
- Conduct problems
- Sleepwalking and sleep talking
- Headache upon awakening

In addition to the psychological and behavioral problems associated with OSA, over time, untreated OSA can lead to a number of physical health conditions, including diabetes, hypertension, and cardiovascular disease. Therefore, early identification and intervention are key in preventing the long-term negative consequences associated with the disorder.

# *Restless Legs Syndrome*

Restless Legs Syndrome (RLS) is a neurological movement disorder that can wreak havoc on sleep. RLS is characterized by an intense and uncomfortable urge to move one's legs while at rest. This irresistible urge to move typically occurs when the child lies down to sleep, but it can occur any time he or she is sitting or lying still. In order to alleviate the discomfort, the child must move his or her legs or get up and walk around. Movement alleviates the discomfort, but only temporarily. The prevalence of RLS in children is around 2 percent, and the disorder has a relatively high comorbidity with ADHD and mood and anxiety disorders (Picchietti & Picchietti, 2008). Following are the diagnostic criteria set forth by the International Restless Legs Syndrome Study Group:

1. An urge to move the legs usually but not always accompanied by or felt to be caused by uncomfortable and unpleasant sensations in the legs

2. The urge to move the legs and any accompanying unpleasant sensations begin or worsen during periods of rest or inactivity such as lying down or sitting
3. The urge to move the legs and any accompanying unpleasant sensations are partially or totally relieved by movement, such as walking or stretching, at least as long as the activity continues
4. The urge to move the legs and any accompanying unpleasant sensations during rest or inactivity only occur or are worse in the evening or night than during the day
5. The above features are not solely accounted for as symptoms primary to another medical or behavioral condition (e.g., myalgia, leg edema, arthritis, leg cramps, habitual foot tapping).
6. As noted above, RLS is a neurological condition, but it has significant negative effects on sleep. For instance, RLS makes it difficult to fall asleep and leads to sleep disruption throughout the

night. Both RLS-related outcomes can lead to significant psychological and behavioral impairment during the day.

# PSYCHOPHARMACOLOGY

## *Pharmacology of Insomnia*

In each instance, the pharmacological approach of choice is not to use sleeping pills, but rather to treat the psychiatric disorder (e.g., with antidepressants, mood stabilizers) that is causing the insomnia. Furthermore, even when treatment specifically for the insomnia is warranted, pharmacotherapy is generally not the recommended first-line approach.

Behavioral interventions have the most research support for both children and adults suffering from insomnia. For example, treatments of choice include no caffeine after 2p.m., proper sleep hygiene (e.g., reducing the amount of intensity during evening hours, including exciting video games and movies), sleeping in a dark and quiet room (with no television in the bedroom), and reduced screen time in the evening. *Screen time* refers to time spent looking at television, computer, and cell phone screens. Research has shown that more than 2 hours a day of screen time is associated with increased rates of psychological symptoms and substance abuse (Campaign for a Commercial-Free Childhood, 2014; see http://www.screenfree.org for a review). Additionally, all screens emit large amounts of blue-wavelength light, which has been shown to suppress the natural melatonin release that begins a couple of hours before sleep, and can thus reduce the quality of sleep. Of interest is the use of amber-colored glasses that are worn in the evening, which selectively screen out blue-wavelength light (these can be easily found on the Internet).

Pharmacological treatments for insomnia include the use of the following medications: sleeping pills (e.g., zaleplon [Sonata], eszopiclone [Lunesta], and zolpidem [Ambien]), benzodiazepines (e.g., Ativan), alpha-2 agonists (e.g., clonidine), antihistamines (e.g., Atarax and Benadryl), and low doses of sedating antidepressants such as Remeron (7.5–15mg), Silenor (3–6mg), and trazodone (25–100mg). Medications for sleep aren't without side effects. For example, some children will actually experience anxiety when treated with trazodone due to the action of metachlorophenylpiperazine (MCPP), which is a metabolic byproduct of trazodone (Brent, 2013). Sleeping pills like Ambien and Lunesta have been tied to amnesia and associated amnestic behavior such as eating, driving, and even sexual behavior without no memory of the event. And antihistamines like Atarax (hydroxyzine hydrochloride) and Benadryl (diphenhydramine) can have a paradoxical effect and lead to excitability and restlessness after taking the medication.

Melatonin, which is a synthetic hormone, is an over-the-counter product commonly used to improve sleep. Recently concerns have been raised by the National Institutes of Health regarding the use of melatonin in children (see chapter 10). However, many prescribers prefer to start with melatonin before moving to medications with more known significant side effects.

Caution is advised in prescribing these drugs except in cases where very short-term treatment is the goal. By and large, the nonmedical approaches listed above are most strongly recommended. Sleep medications tend to lose their effectiveness over time, and they do not address the underlying cause of the insomnia.

A significant number of children do not have a sleep disorder per se, but simply do not sleep enough. Youngsters stay up late often to play video games, watch television, or be on the Internet, social media, or cell phones. But children ages 1 to 5 need 12 to 14 hours of sleep per night; children ages 6 to 12 need 9 to 11 hours; and teenagers need 9 hours per night. Of course, sleep deprivation always results in some degree of daytime fatigue and decreased ability to maintain concentration. However, beyond this is the significant negative impact of reduced sleep on all psychiatric disorders. Gangwisch et al. (2010) conducted an in-home survey on 15,652 adolescents in grades 7 to 12. In particular, they tried to assess the impact of sleep deprivation on rates of depression and suicidal ideation. Subjects were matched for sex, age, ethnicity, and parental marital status. Gangwisch and colleagues compared outcomes for teens who routinely went to bed before 10p.m. to those who routinely went to bed after midnight. Those going to bed at midnight or later showed 24 percent more depression and were 20 percent more likely to have had suicidal ideation during the past 12 months. It should be noted that significantly decreased amounts of slow-wave (deep) sleep can alone result in depression in 40 to 45 percent of people (this can occur in people who have insomnia, sleep apnea, or restless legs). The authors remarked that most adolescents actually do go to bed when told by their parents.

## *Pharmacology of Nightmares*

Similar to insomnia, the effective treatment of nightmares generally requires adequately addressing the underlying cause (e.g., acute or chronic stress, post-traumatic stress disorder, anxiety). For many, resolution of the primary psychiatric disorder will lead to resolution of the nightmares.

When specific targeting of nightmares is required, again, like insomnia, nonpharmacological interventions should be considered first. The psychotherapeutic intervention with the most research support in addressing nightmares is imagery rehearsal therapy (IRT; Ho, Chan, & Tang, 2016). IRT, or similar variants of IRT (e.g., imagery rescripting therapy) consists of psychoeducation about sleep and nightmares and requires the person to change the narrative of his or her dream to a version that is less distressing. The lion's share of research is specific to adults; however, a number of small case reports and uncontrolled studies support the use of IRT with children (Simard & Nielsen, 2009; St-Onge, Mercier, & De Koninck, 2009).

Pharmacological treatments for nightmares in children are similar to those used in adults. These include alpha-1 antagonists (e.g., prazosin) and medications with antihistaminic and serotonergic properties (e.g., cyproheptadine, trazodone; Waltman, Shearer, & Moore, 2018).

It should be noted, however, that there are very little data available on the effective and safe use of medications for the treatment of nightmares in children. Medications should be used only as a last resort and by prescribers with experience using pharmacological agents in children suffering from nightmares.

## *Pharmacology of Obstructive Sleep Apnea and Restless Legs Syndrome*

The pharmacological treatment of OSA is symptom-focused. There is no medication to correct sleep apnea; however, medications can be used to combat daytime fatigue and drowsiness. These include psychostimulants (e.g., Adderall, Ritalin) and other wake-promoting agents (e.g., Provigil,

Nuvigil). The treatment of choice is forced air pressure via an appliance such as a continuous positive airway pressure (CPAP) or automatic positive airway pressure (APAP) device. In milder forms of the disorder, a dental appliance may suffice.

Medications are available to treat RLS and include dopamine agonists (e.g., Mirapex, Requip), benzodiazepines (e.g., Xanax, Klonopin, Restoril) and anticonvulsants (e.g., Neurontin, Horizant). In mild cases, self-care techniques such as taking hot or cold baths, using hot or cold packs, massage, and relaxation techniques may be all that is required. Prevention is also key to managing RLS. Caffeine, nicotine, and medications known to worsen RLS should be avoided. For example, certain antihistamines (e.g., Benadryl, Atarax) and serotonergic antidepressants (e.g., Prozac, Zoloft, Paxil) can exacerbate RLS.

# *Initiating Treatment and Precautions*

The initial choice of medication should be based on the type of symptoms that are interfering most with the child's sleep symptoms, side-effect profile, and wishes of the child and parents or guardians. Once chosen, the medication should be started at a low dose and monitored closely for effects, both positive and negative. It should be noted that there are very little data available for treating any sleep problem with medication. The decision to use medication for insomnia, nightmares, OSA, RLS, or any other sleep complaint should not be made lightly, and the risks and benefits should be weighed carefully. We believe strongly that nonpharmacological interventions should be considered first and medical treatments should be utilized only when nonpharmacological treatments have failed. Furthermore, most medications used for sleep disorders for children are off label, and when medications are prescribed for children suffering from sleep complaints, they should be done so only by those with specific training and experience working with children.

# CHAPTER 9

# Miscellaneous Disorders

In this chapter we will discuss several disorders more briefly.

## SUBSTANCE USE DISORDER

Substance use has been shown to be common during adolescence, prompting widespread public concern. According to a report by the Center on Addiction and Substance Abuse at Columbia University, in 2011 three-quarters of high school students had used addictive substances (e.g., cigarettes, alcohol, marijuana, cocaine). 46 percent of high school students used addictive substances, and 12 percent met the criteria for addiction. Interestingly, a 2011 survey of this group of teenagers ages 12 to 17 who spent significant time on social networking sites (e.g., Facebook) showed that they were five times more likely to use tobacco, three times more likely to have used alcohol, and twice as likely to have used marijuana (Center on Addiction, 2011a, 2011b).

The mainstay of the treatment of substance use disorders in adolescence, as in adults, continues to be nonpharmacological treatment, especially 12-step programs such as Alateen. However, medication can play an important role. It should be noted that medications for substance abuse have been studied almost exclusively in adults, so the suggested uses are based on extrapolation from adult data and must be viewed with caution. Medications can help with the following:

- Treating intoxication (for example, naltrexone for heroin overdose)
- Treating withdrawal states (for example, benzodiazepines for alcohol withdrawal)
- Reducing craving (for example, gabapentin or acamprosate for alcohol)
- Acting as a deterrent (for example, Antabuse for alcohol)
- Treating comorbid psychiatric disorders

# Diagnostic Issues

In *DSM-5,* substance-related disorders are divided into the following categories: substance use disorder, intoxication, and withdrawal. The word *addiction* is no longer used in *DSM;* rather, substance use disorders now are described as ranging from mild to severe. In addition, each substance may have related disorders phenomenologically similar to other disorders: delirium; dementia; and amnestic, psychotic, mood, anxiety, sexual, and sleep disorders.

*Substance use* is defined in *DSM-5* as a pattern of substance use leading to significant impairment or distress, demonstrated by at least three of the following:

- Tolerance, as shown by either diminished effect with use of the same amount or a need for markedly increased amounts. Depending on the individual's use pattern and genetic makeup, tolerance can develop quickly or more slowly, over months or years.

- Withdrawal, which is a physiological process in which the body "craves" continued use of the substance. The substance is often used more than was intended and in situations that are increasingly problematic (e.g., at school, while alone at home).
- A persistent desire or unsuccessful efforts to cut down or control substance use. This is often in conflict with the adolescent's verbal reassurance that he or she can quit or cut down on the amount used if desired.
- A great deal of time spent obtaining the substance. This often manifests in neglecting school, work, or family obligations.
- Giving up or reducing participation in important social, occupational, or recreational activities because of substance use. This often occurs due to rejection from peers who do not use substances and/or comorbid depression or anxiety.
- Continued substance use despite having a problem that is likely to have been caused or exacerbated by the substance. This can be a

physical (health), psychological, financial, or interpersonal problem.

Severe substance use disorders are often characterized by the following:

- Recurrent substance use resulting in a failure to fulfill obligations at work, school, or home.
- Recurrent substance use in situations in which it is physically hazardous (for example, driving an automobile or operating a machine when impaired by substance use).
- Recurrent substance-related legal problems (for example, driving while impaired, "minor in possession," etc.).
- Continued substance use despite having persistent or recurrent social or interpersonal problems caused or exacerbated by the effects of the substance.

*Intoxication* refers to an acutely altered mental state due to ingestion of, or exposure to, a substance. This is a potentially dangerous condition in which substance toxicity can lead to reduced respiration or heart rate, and overall central nervous system depression.

*Withdrawal* refers to an altered state produced by cessation or reduction of use of a substance that causes significant impairment in functioning in important areas. The disorder may be "persisting"; in other words, it may continue even though substance use has stopped and the withdrawal syndrome has been resolved.

| SUBSTANCES WITH THE POTENTIAL FOR ABUSE | | | | | |
|---|---|---|---|---|---|
| **Substance** | **Dependence** | **Abuse** | **Intoxication** | **Withdrawal** | **Persisting** |
| Alcohol | X | X | X | X | X |
| Hallucinogens | X | X | X | | X |
| Opioids | X | X | X | X | |
| Phencyclidine (PCP) | X | X | X | | |
| Sedative-hypnotics | X | X | X | X | X |
| Stimulants | X | X | X | X | X |
| Cannabis | X | X | X | X | |

Figure 8-A

## MAJOR SUBSTANCE DIAGNOSES

**Alcohol.** Alcohol (ethanol) is a water-soluble substance that is rapidly absorbed and readily crosses the blood–brain barrier. It is a central nervous system (CNS) depressant and is metabolized by the liver, in addition to being a gastric irritant and toxic to liver cells and neurons. Alcohol is probably the most studied substance of abuse (and the most abused substance). It is associated with dependence, abuse, withdrawal, intoxication, delirium, dementia, amnesia, delusions, hallucinations, depression, anxiety, sexual dysfunction, and sleep problems. Much evidence demonstrates that alcoholism is familial, but the exact biological mechanism remains unclear.

Psychiatric symptoms are very common in alcohol intoxication and withdrawal, especially anxiety and depression. Often these symptoms will resolve within a few weeks without any pharmacological treatment. However, medications can play an important role in the treatment of alcohol-related disorders. Most of these medications are discussed elsewhere in this book, but a few are specific to alcoholism treatment. Disulfiram (Antabuse) is a medication used in abstinence maintenance. Antabuse causes an accumulation of acetaldehyde if a person drinks alcohol while taking it, which leads to an unpleasant and potentially dangerous reaction involving flushing, throbbing headache, nausea, and vomiting. Antabuse treatment is only appropriate for certain people. Some are able to remain abstinent without it; some will drink despite taking it. In between are those who will be able to reinforce their desire for abstinence by taking 125 to 500mg of disulfiram once daily. Antabuse should be used with caution because of its toxicity with alcohol and in overdose. It should be used in the treatment of adolescents only when they are under close supervision and when there is a relatively strong belief that the adolescent can remain abstinent. Two other medications have been shown to help in abstinence maintenance by reducing craving: naltrexone, an opiate antagonist, has shown some promise (Bender, 1993); and acamprosate (Campral), a GABA-receptor agonist, has been recently released to aid in abstinence maintenance. Campral has been shown to be safe and well tolerated, but it does require dosing three times daily.

**Stimulants.** Amphetamines, ecstasy, and cocaine have become common substances of abuse. They are CNS stimulants that act on the dopaminergic system. Research suggests that a dopamine-mediated endogenous reward circuit in the limbic system is activated by amphetamines and cocaine. This means that use of these drugs is intensely pleasurable, hence their addictiveness.

Pharmacological treatment of stimulant use is different for each phase of use. During acute intoxication, medications such as benzodiazepines, beta-blockers, and clonidine can be used to block the acute effects of dopamine and norepinephrine (to control anxiety, heart rate, and blood pressure and prevent seizures). During withdrawal, medications such as antidepressants and amantadine are used to reduce craving (and hopefully subsequent use).

**Opiates.** Heroin was first synthesized from morphine over a century ago. Since then, it has become one of the most abused substances.

Research into the reasons it produces such powerful effects has led to the discovery of specific opiate receptors and endogenous opioids (enkephalins and endorphins). These peptides appear to be neurotransmitters involved with the sensations of pain and pleasure. In clinical practice, opiates are used primarily as analgesics. A number of the available opiates can lead to dependency, including morphine, heroin, methadone, meperidine (Demerol), pentazocine, hydromorphone (Dilaudid), oxycodone (Percocet, Oxycontin), hydrocodone (Vicodin, Norco, Lorcet, Lortab), and codeine. It should be noted that opiate-abuse trends among adolescents are not the use of heroin or methadone, but rather readily available prescription opiates (Percocet, Vicodin), which are found in many home medicine cabinets across the country. Young athletes who are more likely to experience physical injuries and subsequent pain are particularly at increased risk due to the need to manage acute or chronic pain at such an early age.

Different medications are used to treat different phases of opiate use. Acute opiate intoxication leads to sedation, pupillary constriction, and respiratory depression and can be fatal. Specific antagonists—naloxone and naltrexone—block the opiate receptors and rapidly (and sometimes dramatically) reverse these effects. Opiate withdrawal is characterized by anxiety, agitation, sweating, gastrointestinal (GI) upset, tremulousness, and running nose. It is treated by using another opiate, such as methadone, or clonidine, or a combination of these. Dependence or abuse can be treated using one of two strategies. One is to administer methadone, a long-acting synthetic opiate that is well tolerated and reduces craving for other opiates such as heroin. Methadone is used for maintenance treatment because, with its long half-life, it produces less of a "high" and is less prone to abuse. The other is to use an opiate antagonist (naloxone, naltrexone), or a mixed opioid agonist–antagonist like buprenorphine) so the effect of the opiate will be blocked if it is used.

**Hallucinogens.** Various substances can produce transient psychotic states, often accompanied by visual, auditory, or olfactory hallucinations. These include LSD, mescaline, psilocybin, and PCP. These drugs are not associated with dependence or withdrawal, but they can produce florid psychosis during acute intoxication. This effect can be allowed to run its course (usually 12 to 24 hours), but sometimes medications, such as antianxiety or antipsychotic drugs, need to be used to decrease agitation and stabilize blood pressure. Severe overdoses of PCP can lead to convulsions and may require emergency medical treatment.

**Marijuana and other drugs.** Marijuana (cannabis) was not previously considered a drug that would produce tolerance, dependence, and abuse. However—possibly because forms of marijuana popular today may have up to ten times the THC (delta-9-tetrahydrocannabinol) content of the marijuana of the 1970s (Brangham, 2014)—it is now recognized that cannabis use may lead to dependence, abuse, intoxication, delirium, psychotic disorder, mood disorder, and anxiety disorder. Cannabis usually produces dependence because of its calming effect. Prolonged use leads to what has been called an *amotivational syndrome,* associated with decreased initiative, activity, and energy. In some individuals, paradoxically, intoxication may lead to anxiety, and even psychosis (see sidebar below). Withdrawal is usually associated with anxiety symptoms and occasionally paranoia. There are no specific treatments for cannabis-induced disorders. However, antianxiety medications are used for anxiety symptoms and antipsychotics are administered for psychotic symptoms. Contrary to popular belief among proponents of cannabis use for psychiatric disorders (e.g., post-traumatic stress disorder, anxiety), there is little credible evidence to support its use for this purpose.

Other substances of abuse, including nicotine, inhalants, and caffeine, are not covered here since their psychiatric effects are less important in a clinical setting.

## Cannabis: Relaxation, Anxiety, Mania, and Psychosis

Cannabis contains a number of biologically active molecules, including two important psychoactive compounds: CBD (cannabidiol) and THC (delta-9-tetrahydrocannabinol). CBD activates cannabinoid receptors in a number of brain regions, including the amygdala. Here it reduces metabolic activity and calms anxiety. However, THC has been associated with the ignition of mania in people who have bipolar disorder, and may provoke an earlier onset of psychotic episodes in those destined to develop schizophrenia (DiForti et al., 2009; Lynch, Rabin, & George, 2012). This mix of neurological actions can, in a *seemingly* paradoxical manner, either reduce anxiety or provoke significant psychiatric symptoms. How this affects any one individual may have to do with unique personal sensitivities or the relative concentrations of CBD and

THC. Whether cannabis is legal or not, there are physical and psychological health risks.

## TIC DISORDERS AND TOURETTE SYNDROME

Tourette (or Gilles de la Tourette) syndrome (TS) affects an estimated 0.3 to 0.8 percent of children and is characterized by motor and vocal tics—sudden involuntary movements or vocalizations. TS is known most for coprolalia (sudden yelling of obscenities), but this symptom is seen in only 25 to 30 percent of cases and is not as severe as is often noted in television or movie portrayals of the condition. Motor tics typically involve the head and neck. Vocal tics may be guttural sounds, repeated coughing, sniffling or snorting, or words. TS was originally viewed as a psychological disorder, but in light of its responsiveness to medications, especially dopamine blockers, this view has changed. Although symptoms may be exacerbated by anxiety or tension, TS is now generally considered to be a neurological disorder that appears to involve dysfunction of dopaminergic pathways. TS is usually treated with dopamine (D2) blockers—haloperidol or pimozide, in low to moderate doses; or, more recently, risperidone. Children with TS have a higher incidence of obsessive-compulsive disorder (OCD), attention-deficit/hyperactivity disorder (ADHD), and learning disorders (Stern et al., 2000), probably because TS can involve multiple areas of the brain, some of which are also associated with OCD and ADHD. Theories regarding the etiology of TS include genetic (Robertson & Stern, 1997) and autoimmune mechanisms related to strep infection (Bowes, 2001).

## *Diagnostic Issues*

The diagnosis of Tourette syndrome according to *DSM-5* is based on the following criteria:

- Both motor (multiple) and vocal (one or more) tics have been present at some time during the

illness, although not necessarily concurrently.
- The tics come and go, but have been present for more than 1 year.
- The onset is before age 18.
- The tics are not the direct result of a substance (illicit or prescribed) or another medical condition.

## *Psychopharmacology*

Using medication to reduce the intensity and frequency of tics may not be necessary and should not be considered an essential part of treatment. The goal of pharmacotherapy should be to suppress tics to a tolerable level, not to eliminate tics. Often, treatment of comorbid disorders, such as OCD or ADHD, is more important. When the tics are of sufficient severity that they are very embarrassing or interfere with other activities, pharmacological treatment should be considered. If left untreated, significant socialization problems can arise, as can mood and anxiety issues. The mainstays of treatment for tic suppression are the dopamine blockers (first-generation antipsychotics), such as haloperidol, pimozide, and perphenazine. Haloperidol has been widely used, but pimozide and perphenazine have fewer side effects. Although these medications are very effective in tic suppression, their neuroleptic side effects make them poorly tolerated. Although not approved by the FDA for treatment of TS, Risperdal (a second-generation antipsychotic) is now seen as a preferred treatment by some (Walkup, 2004) and shown to be equally effective as haloperidol and pimozide (Eddy & Rickards, 2011). After adequate tic suppression is achieved, stimulants can be added for comorbid ADHD, or selective serotonin reuptake inhibitors (SSRIs) can be added for comorbid OCD. It is usually better to use the lowest dose sufficient to reduce tics than to use a higher dose to try to eliminate tics. These medications and their side effects are discussed in detail in chapter 5.

The alpha-adrenergic agonists clonidine and guanfacine represent another type of medication that has shown effectiveness. These medications were developed as antihypertensives and therefore may cause a severe drop in blood pressure. Because they also have some benefit in the treatment of ADHD, they may be most helpful in cases with comorbid ADHD, or when the dopamine blockers are not tolerated. Treatment with clonidine usually begins with 0.025 to 0.05mg per day and increases slowly to 0.1 to 0.3mg per day in two to four divided doses. Children should be monitored for sedation and low blood pressure. Guanfacine, though less studied, may cause less sedation, require less-frequent dosing, and have more impact on attention because of its preferential binding at prefrontal cortical regions and its longer half-life.

# EATING DISORDERS

Eating disorders, which are fairly common in adolescents, can result in significant medical complications. There are three main types of eating disorders: anorexia nervosa, bulimia nervosa, and binge-eating disorder.

Anorexia involves the maintenance of a very low body weight by restriction of intake, purging, or both, often in combination with excessive exercising. Anorexia can be fatal, usually due to cardiac complications. Bulimia involves repeated episodes of bingeing and purging: eating large amounts of food and then purging through self-induced vomiting or use of laxatives or diuretics. It can lead to significant dental disease or GI bleeding. Binge-eating disorder refers to consuming large amounts of food without purging. It leads to obesity.

## *Diagnostic Issues*

For anorexia nervosa, the diagnostic criteria are as follows:

- Food intake restriction leading to significantly low body weight
- Intense fear of gaining weight or becoming "fat," despite being underweight
- Distortion of body image (perceiving oneself as overweight when actually underweight)

For bulimia nervosa, diagnostic criteria are as follows:

- Recurrent episodes of binge eating, characterized by eating large amounts of food while feeling out of control
- Use of compensatory behavior to prevent weight gain, such as self-induced vomiting or misuse of laxatives or diuretics
- Binge eating and compensatory behaviors both occurring an average of at least once a week for 3 months

For binge-eating disorder, diagnostic criteria are as follows

- Excessive eating during a discrete time period (e.g., 1–2 hours)
- Feeling a lack of control over eating, often accompanied by:
    - Eating rapidly
    - Eating until feeling uncomfortably full
    - Eating when not feeling hungry
    - Feeling guilt, shame, embarrassment, or disgust at oneself for overeating

- Unlike bulimia nervosa, there is not compensatory behavior (such as purging or use of laxatives)

## *Psychopharmacology*

Much research has investigated personality characteristics, psychological issues, family dynamics, and the biological bases of these eating disorders. Anorexia usually requires a multimodal, if not multidisciplinary, treatment approach. The severe nutritional deficiency from anorexia causes a multitude of problems that must be addressed medically and make response to medication treatment alone poor. Indeed, no medication has shown significant consistent benefit in the treatment of anorexia, with the possible exception of atypical antipsychotics. It is known that endorphins are released during prolonged fasting; one theory suggests that patients with anorexia become addicted to starvation, and that anorexics have a biological vulnerability to this addiction. Studies have shown some benefit from naltrexone (an opiate antagonist) in the treatment of anorexia—the explanation being that it blocks the "high" of fasting and thereby removes the incentive (Luby, Marrazzi, & Kinzie, 1987). Other medications that are *sometimes* helpful include antidepressants, antipsychotics, cyproheptadine, lithium, and anticonvulsants. These drugs can be especially useful in cases with coexisting features—antidepressants when depressive symptoms are present, for example.

Patients with bulimia, in contrast, often benefit from treatment with antidepressants (40 to 70 percent respond); this disorder is considered by some to be a depressive variant. All types of antidepressants have proven useful, although it should be remembered that bupropion (Wellbutrin) is contraindicated in eating disorders because of increased risk of seizures. SSRIs have been quite effective and, because of their low side-effect profile, are the most widely used treatment.

The pharmacological treatment of binge-eating disorder is still under investigation and unclear in children, although there are reports that, like bulimia, it often responds to treatment with antidepressants, metformin (an antidiabetes drug), or Topamax (an anticonvulsant). Furthermore, the psychostimulant lisdexamfetamine (Vyvanse) is FDA approved for moderate to severe binge-eating disorder in adults (Heo & Duggan, 2017) and may be effective for adolescents as well (although there is little to no credible research supporting this notion).

# CONDUCT DISORDER

The most important point we wish to make regarding conduct disorder (CD) is that the outward signs of aggression, antisocial behavior, and disregard for social rules that characterize it are often seen in the context of other primary psychiatric disorders. A common mistake with apparent diagnoses of CD is failure to diagnose an underlying and potentially treatable primary disorder. It is thus critical to conduct a comprehensive assessment to determine whether there is an underlying psychiatric disorder, especially one of the following:

significant situational stress, bipolar disorder, major depression, ADHD, emotional dyscontrol secondary to neurological injury (seen in some children who have sustained closed-head injuries, for example), or substance abuse. The only pharmacological treatments used for pure CD target aggression, irritability, and impulsivity. These medications include atypical antipsychotics (such as risperidone), clonidine, and SSRIs. The selection of a medication depends on the child's health and psychiatric history and unique symptom presentation.

# ENURESIS AND ENCOPRESIS

Enuresis and encopresis are considered elimination disorders as they involve the inappropriate elimination (in bed or clothes) of urine and feces. Enuresis (inappropriate elimination of urine) generally begins in childhood. Some inappropriate elimination of urine is expected in younger children (aged 5 or less); however, as the child matures, continued inappropriate intentional or unintentional urination may be a sign of a psychological or medical problem. Enuresis has three variations: nocturnal (during sleep), diurnal (during waking hours), and nocturnal and diurnal. The first-line treatment of nocturnal enuresis is the use of a moisture-sensitive pad with an alarm that fits under bedding. If this method is not successful, or if the child experiences diurnal enuresis, the tricyclic antidepressant imipramine (Tofranil) may be used. Other medications shown to be helpful are desmopressin acetate and anticholinergics (e.g., oxybutynin).

Encopresis (elimination of feces) also generally begins in childhood and is the elimination of feces in inappropriate places (e.g., clothes, floor). As with enuresis, some inappropriate elimination of feces is expected in young children. However, if it continues after the age of 4 or 5, this may be a sign of a psychological or physical condition. Since encopresis is often related to constipation, dietary and colon cleansing may be all that is required. In some cases, the use of laxatives may be required along with behavioral modification.

# CHAPTER 10

# Over-the-Counter Medications and Dietary Supplements

In the United States each year, people spend $500 million for over-the-counter (OTC) herbal remedies and dietary supplements that purport to treat psychiatric disorders. There are a number of reasons that many people choose these products rather than seeking more traditional medical solutions. These reasons include wanting to use only "natural" medications, fearing that standard FDA-approved pharmaceuticals may be habit-forming or likely to cause serious side effects, needing to find treatments that are less expensive than prescription drugs, and desiring to seek relief from psychiatric symptoms without consulting a mental health professional or personal physician (this is largely about the negative stigma associated with treatment for mental illnesses). Additionally, many patients seeking psychotherapy may already be taking such OTC drugs when they enter therapy, and many will have questions regarding the efficacy and safety of these products.

During the past two decades, there has been a significant increase in the number of patients seeking complementary and alternative medicine (CAM). Recent surveys show that up to 40 percent of Americans have turned to CAM for the treatment of many illnesses. Mood-altering agents such as Saint-John's-wort and SAM-e are among the top-selling dietary supplements. It is important to be aware that 70 percent of people taking these products never mention them to their physician. At times this can be very problematic—especially as it relates to drug–drug interactions.

There are several OTC products that have been shown to be effective in treating depression and anxiety. These are reviewed in this chapter. (Note that many OTC products have been suggested to have indications in the treatment of psychiatric disorders, but we are only including those that have the strongest empirical evidence.) First, however, it is important to address three concerns. One is that many individuals prefer to be treated with something that is "natural," assuming that natural also means "safe." This is not always the case. Some OTC products are well known for producing significant (and sometimes dangerous) drug–drug interactions, most notably Saint-John's-wort. This herbal product has complex effects on liver metabolism, inhibiting some liver enzymes and inducing others, which can lead to a number of potentially serious drug–drug interactions.

Second, the FDA does not have oversight of dietary supplements. Many of these products are not quality controlled. There have been numerous cases in which some products did not contain the advertised amount of the drug or contained impurities or contaminants (e.g., lead, mercury, arsenic). A 2013 study investigated forty-four OTC products from dozens of companies. Of the products tested, 50 percent contained plant species not listed on the bottle, and 30 percent had absolutely none of the plant listed on the bottle (in fact, one product reported to be Saint-John's-wort only contained a plant that was an herbal laxative). With no standardization requirements, consumers have no way to determine if the product they buy is safe or if it contains the actual ingredient at the advertised dose/potency. Three organizations—US Pharmacopeia (USP), NSF International, and Consumerlab.co m—independently evaluate OTC drugs and dietary supplements. If USP's or NSF's insignia is printed on the bottle, or if the product is appropriately verified on Consumerlab.com, customers can be assured that the product they are buying is the real thing at the potency listed on the bottle and that it is free of contaminants. These organizations, however, do not evaluate efficacy, and neither does the Food and Drug Administration.

A third and very important issue is that generally these products are purchased and taken without medical supervision. People self-diagnose and then take the medications or supplement. At times this can lead to disaster. This is especially true when people have undiagnosed bipolar disorder and begin taking Saint-John's-wort, 5-HTP, or SAM-e, all of which have been shown to reduce depressive symptoms. An individual may experience significant depressive symptoms, assume they represent garden-variety depression, and take an OTC product, perhaps even treating his or her children. Within 3 to 5 weeks, the drug can provoke switching into a manic episode. It is well known that any treatment that reduces depressive symptoms can potentially provoke manic episodes in people who have bipolar disorder. In a number of countries where there is widespread use of herbal and dietary supplements to treat psychiatric disorders, there are also strong incentives for people to first be carefully diagnosed by a physician or other mental health professional and then be followed and monitored by a physician as the treatment begins. For example, in Germany, dietary and herbal supplements are available over-the-counter for purchase; however, if the patient is evaluated and treated by a physician, he or she receives a prescription and the medicine at no cost (paid for by the government). Those who want to take OTC drugs should be carefully evaluated and followed by a physician or a mental health expert.

# OVER-THE-COUNTER OPTIONS FOR TREATING DEPRESSION

It should be noted that to date, almost none of the following products have been subject to randomized controlled trials with children, and thus safety and efficacy have not been carefully evaluated for use with children. The one exception is omega-3 fatty acids. Five OTC products have research support for efficacy in treating depression in adults and older adolescents: Saint-John's-wort, SAM-e, 5-HTP, omega-3 fatty acids, and folic acid. The first three of these have been used to treat depression as a stand-alone monotherapy. Folic acid and omega-3 fatty acids are used to augment antidepressants. Summarized below is information regarding dosing and side effects for each of these products. As side effects are discussed, keep in mind that all of these products (except omega-3 fatty acids and folic acid) can provoke mania in bipolar patients.

## *Saint-John's-Wort*

In a meta-analysis of studies evaluating the efficacy of Saint-John's-wort, this drug has treatment outcomes showing it to be equally effective as prescription antidepressants (Linde, Berner, & Kriston, 2008). It is well tolerated, with side effects including mild nausea and sometimes photosensitivity (sensitivity to sunburns). In order to treat severe depression, the doses need to be high (i.e., 1,500–1,800mg per day). Treatment should begin at 300mg a day and over a period of 2 weeks titrate up to 1,500 or 1,800mg a day. These higher doses require three-times-a-day dosing to avoid nausea and other GI symptoms, which would occur if the daily dose were to be taken all at once. As noted above, drug–drug interactions can be problematic and sometimes dangerous. It is best to check with a pharmacist who can review all of the patient's medications to determine if adverse interactions are likely to occur.

## *SAM-e*

SAM-e (S-adenosylmethionine) is a naturally occurring biomolecule. Meta-analyses show it to be equally effective as standard antidepressants (Williams, Girard, Jui, Sabina, & Katz, 2005). Most people who take SAM-e experience no side effects, but side effects do occur and can include nausea, diarrhea, headaches, restlessness, and insomnia. SAM-e should never be given with MAOIs (monoamine oxidase inhibitors), which can cause a serotonin syndrome (dangerous and sometimes fatal). Doses required to treat severe depression need to be between 800 and 1,600mg a day.

# *Omega-3 Fatty Acids*

Omega-3 fatty acids have shown promise as an augmenting agent in the treatment of depression. They are superior to placebo as an augmenting medication. There are several types of omega-3 fatty acids: linolenic acid (derived from flaxseed, chia seed, and walnut oil), EPA, and DHA (the latter two are from fish oil). A good deal of research has revealed that fatty acids from fish oil or krill are significantly more bioavailable in the brain than those derived from nut and seed oils. Thus, linolenic acid has little effect in the brain. Additionally, EPA is the specific omega-3 fatty acid that appears to have an impact on depression and irritability. "Omega-3 fatty acids in particular have a strong record of safety, compelling rationale for use in bipolar disorder, and have already been shown to have significant preventive effects in decreasing the transition from early symptoms to full-blown schizophrenia," according to Post (2013). In addition, omega-3 fatty acids afford slight improvement in children with ADHD.

It is important to note that upon close inspection of the product label, many fish oil products have relatively small amounts of EPA. In the studies where omega-3 is effective in treating depression, for example, the amount of EPA required to produce positive results is 1,000 to 2,000mg (1 to 2 grams). Few OTC preparations of fish oil contain this much EPA. Omega-3 at these doses is very well tolerated, with few side effects. It can produce some mild GI upset.

## *5-HTP*

5-HTP, which is derived from the amino acid tryptophan, is an effective and well tolerated antidepressant (one used frequently in Japan). It has been shown to be effective for major depression (Shaw, Turner, & Del Mar, 2002). Typical dosing is 300mg a day, and this can be increased to 600mg a day. At times 5-HTP can cause serotonin syndrome, and it should not be given with prescription antidepressants that work via increasing serotonin levels in the brain.

## *Folic Acid*

Folic acid has been shown to be an effective augmenting drug when added to antidepressants (Taylor, Carney, Geddes, & Goodwin, 2003). The typical dose is 400–800 mcg per day, and at these doses there are generally no side effects. If a patient is being treated with Depakote, higher doses of folic acid are required because Depakote depletes folate. The recommended dose in this case is 1mg a day for females and 2mg a day for males.

# OTHER OTC PRODUCTS

The research database for the following products is scant. However, the following may be options for treating certain target symptoms.

## *Melatonin for Treatment of Sleep Disorders*

Melatonin is a naturally occurring hormone produced in the pineal gland in the brain. It helps to promote deep sleep. One of melatonin's effects is to help to cool the body down during sleep, which facilitates entry into slow-wave (deep) sleep.

In pharmacies and grocery stores, synthetic melatonin can be purchased. During the past 10 years, this product has been widely used as a sleeping pill for children and teenagers. However, recent studies suggest that melatonin may be problematic for use in children, especially at doses of 1–5mg or more. Such doses increase the melatonin in a person's system by a factor of one to twenty times the normal amount. This caution is echoed by both the National Institutes of Health and the National Sleep Foundation: "Melatonin should not be used in most children. It is possibly unsafe. Because of its effects on other hormones, melatonin might interfere with development during adolescence" (National Institutes of Health, 2014). Doses above 0.5mg can aggravate depression and bipolar disorder. It is also important to note that the use of birth control pills can raise levels of melatonin.

Melatonin is, however, sometimes used to treat sleep problems in children who have primary sleep disorders, severe ADHD, and other neurodevelopmental disorders. A low-dose strategy—0.5mg three hours prior to sleep—may be useful in promoting better quality sleep without adverse effects. Melatonin should not be used as a sleeping pill because at this low dose, it does not produce sedation. If higher doses are given, sedation will occur, but this is where melatonin levels may become unsafe. Higher doses can cause drowsiness and may increase depression. The low-dose strategy is recommended.

Melatonin is not habit-forming and is well tolerated. However, it must be noted that the use of melatonin is experimental, so parents should first talk with their pediatrician.

## *Chamomile Tea for Treatment of Anxiety*

One study demonstrated that daily use of chamomile for a period of four weeks can effectively treat generalized anxiety disorder (Amsterdam et al., 2009). In the study, symptomatic improvement was seen when subjects consumed between 200 and 600mg a day. It is difficult to know how many milligrams of chamomile are found in a cup of tea, but it is estimated that a 6-ounce cup of chamomile tea contains 400–600mg. Some people respond to doses as high as 1,500mg per day. Chamomile tea has few side effects. The most common is sedation.

## *Valerian*

Valerian has been used since the days of Hippocrates as a tranquilizer and a sedative-hypnotic. Doses used to treat insomnia are 300–900mg. The mechanism of action is not well understood, but valerian is hypothesized to interact with GABA/benzodiazepine receptors and may be habit-forming in people who are prone to substance abuse.

Please keep in mind that these OTC products lack solid research addressing safety and efficacy in children. It is important to remember that lack of negative research, regulation, or governmental warnings does not equal safety. These products can have significant negative consequences and interfere with a child's physical and psychological development. If OTC options for mood, anxiety, and/or sleep are preferred, it is still important to talk with the child's health care provider. This is particularly true for those children already taking medications or OTC supplements and those on special diets.

# APPENDIX

# Patient and Caregiver Information Sheets on Psychiatric Medications

# PATIENT AND CAREGIVER INFORMATION ON ANTIDEPRESSANTS

The name of your medication is ________________.

IMPORTANT NOTE: The following information is intended to supplement, not substitute for, the expertise and judgment of your physician, pharmacist, or other health care professional. It is not intended to imply that use of the drug is safe, appropriate, or effective for you. It is limited and general—in other words, it is not all-inclusive. Not all uses, side effects, precautions, or drug interactions are listed. Your doctor or pharmacist will provide you with official patient information that is more complete and detailed. Consult your health care professional before using this drug.

## *Uses*

SSRIs and other more recently developed antidepressants such as Effexor, Remeron, and Cymbalta are used in the treatment of a number of disorders, including major depressive disorder, depression associated with manic-depressive illness (bipolar disorder), obsessive-compulsive disorder, panic disorder, generalized anxiety disorder, eating disorders, social anxiety disorder, post-traumatic stress disorder, and premenstrual changes in mood. The antidepressant Wellbutrin is an effective antidepressant, but is generally not used to treat anxiety or eating disorders. These drugs have also been found to be effective in the treatment of several other disorders, including mild depression, separation anxiety disorder, and impulsive or aggressive behavior, although they are not currently approved for these indications.

The doctor may choose to prescribe this medication for a reason not listed here. If you are not sure why this medication is being prescribed, please ask the doctor.

## *How to Use*

Take as directed, usually once a day by mouth. Some side effects, such as nausea, may be reduced by taking the medication with food. It is best to take it at about the same time each day. The dosage is based on your medical condition and response to therapy.

## *Missed Dose*

If you miss a dose, take it as soon as you remember. However, if it is near the time of the next dose, or the next day, skip the missed dose and resume your usual dosing schedule. *Do not double the dose in order to catch up.*

## *Side Effects*

*Side effects occur, to some degree, with all medications. They are usually not serious and do not occur in all individuals. They may sometimes occur before beneficial effects of the medication are noticed. Most side effects will decrease or disappear with time. If a side effect persists, speak to the doctor about appropriate treatment.*

Common side effects that you should report to the doctor at the next appointment include drowsiness and fatigue; anxiety or nervousness, including problems sleeping; headache; nausea or heartburn; muscle tremor; twitching; changes in sex drive or sexual performance; blurred vision; dry mouth; nightmares; and loss of appetite.

Tell your doctor immediately if any of the following unlikely but serious side effects occurs: soreness of the mouth, gums, or throat; skin rash or itching; swelling of the face; any unusual bruising or bleeding; nausea; vomiting; loss of appetite; fatigue; weakness; fever or flu-like symptoms; yellow tinge of the eyes or skin; dark-colored urine; inability to pass urine; tingling in the hands and feet; severe muscle twitching; severe agitation or restlessness; *a switch in mood to an unusual state of happiness, excitement, or irritability, or a marked disturbance in sleep;* or thoughts of suicide or hostility (in rare instances this medication has been associated with suicidal or hostile thoughts; although these thoughts may be seen as a part of the disorder, you should definitely discuss these kinds of thoughts with your doctor).

Report any other side effects not listed above to your physician.

## *Drug Interactions*

Because SSRIs can change the effects of other medication or may be affected by other medication, always check with the doctor or pharmacist before taking any other drugs, including over-the-counter medications such as cold remedies. Inform all doctors and dentists who examine or treat you that you are taking an antidepressant drug.

## *PRECAUTIONS*

- Before taking this medication, tell your doctor or pharmacist if you know you are allergic to it or if you have any other allergies.
- Do not increase or decrease your dose without consulting your doctor.
- This drug may make you dizzy or drowsy; use caution when engaging in activities requiring alertness, such as riding a bike, driving, or using machinery.
- Avoid alcoholic beverages.
- Avoid excessive amounts of caffeine.

- Do not stop taking this medication suddenly, as this may result in withdrawal symptoms such as muscle aches, chills, tingling in your hands or feet, nausea, vomiting, and dizziness.
- All antidepressants can increase the likelihood of seizures. Because of this risk, bupropion (Wellbutrin), in particular, should not be used by persons with bulimia.
- *If you have any questions regarding this medication, do not hesitate to contact the doctor, pharmacist, or nurse.*

# PATIENT AND CAREGIVER INFORMATION ON ANTIANXIETY MEDICATIONS

The name of your medication is ___________.

IMPORTANT NOTE: The following information is intended to supplement, not substitute for, the expertise and judgment of your physician, pharmacist, or other health care professional. It is not intended to imply that use of the drug is safe, appropriate, or effective for you. It is limited and general information—in other words, it is not all-inclusive. Not all uses, side effects, precautions, or drug interactions are listed. Your doctor or pharmacist will provide you with official patient information that is more complete and detailed. Consult your health care professional before using this drug.

## *Uses*

Antianxiety medications can help relieve the symptoms of anxiety but will not alter its cause. In usually prescribed doses, they help to calm and sedate the individual; in higher doses, these drugs may be used to induce sleep. These medications, known as benzodiazepines, may also be used as a muscle relaxant, to treat agitation, to suppress seizures, and prior to some diagnostic procedures or surgery.

The doctor may choose to use this medication for a reason not listed here. If you are not sure why this medication is being prescribed, please ask the doctor.

## *How to Use*

Anxiolytics can reduce agitation and induce calm or sedation usually within an hour. Depending on the medication, they may be taken up to three or four times per day.

## *Missed Dose*

Often this type of medication is taken on a PRN, or as needed, basis. However, if you have been instructed to take the medication on a regular basis, you may wait until the next scheduled time if you miss a dose. *Do not double the dose in order to catch up.*

## Side Effects

*Side effects occur, to some degree, with all medications. They are usually not serious and do not occur in all individuals. They may sometimes occur before beneficial effects of the medication are noticed. Most side effects will decrease or disappear with time. If a side effect persists, speak to the doctor about appropriate treatment.*

Common side effects that should be reported to the doctor at the next appointment include drowsiness and fatigue, loss of coordination, weakness or dizziness, forgetfulness, memory lapses, slurred speech, nausea, and heartburn.

Tell your doctor immediately if any of the following unlikely but serious side effects occurs: disorientation; confusion; worsening of memory; difficulty learning new things; blackouts; amnesia; nervousness, restlessness, excitement, or any other behavior changes; loss of coordination leading to falls; or skin rash.

This type of medication may impair the mental and physical abilities required for driving a car or riding a bike. Avoid these activities if you feel drowsy or slowed down.

Do not stop taking the drug suddenly, especially if you have been on the medication for a number of months or have been taking high doses. Benzodiazepines need to be reduced gradually in order to prevent withdrawal reactions.

Report any other side effects not listed above to your physician.

## *Drug Interactions*

Because antianxiety medications may be affected by other medication, always check with the doctor or pharmacist before taking any other medications, including over-the-counter medication such as cold remedies, especially those that are sedating. Inform all doctors and dentists who examine or treat you that you are taking an antianxiety medication.

# *PRECAUTIONS*

- Before taking this medication, tell your doctor or pharmacist if you know you are allergic to it or if you have any other allergies.
- Do not increase or decrease your dose without consulting your doctor.
- *If you have any questions regarding this medication, do not hesitate to contact the doctor, pharmacist, or nurse.*

# PATIENT AND CAREGIVER INFORMATION ON ANTICONVULSANT MOOD STABILIZERS

The name of your medication is ____________.

IMPORTANT NOTE: The following information is intended to supplement, not substitute for, the expertise and judgment of your physician, pharmacist, or other health care professional. It is not intended to imply that use of the drug is safe, appropriate, or effective for you. It is limited and general—in other words, it is not all-inclusive. Not all uses, side effects, precautions, or drug interactions are listed. Your doctor or pharmacist will provide you with official patient information that is more complete and detailed. Consult your health care professional before using this drug.

## *Common Drug Names*

(Brand and generic)

| | |
|---|---|
| Depakote | (divalproex) |

| | |
|---|---|
| Depakene | (valproic acid) |
| Tegretol, Equetro | (carbamazepine) |

## *Uses*

These medications can be used to treat bipolar disorder, but they are used primarily to treat seizure disorders.

## *How to Use*

Anticonvulsant mood stabilizers are available in different strengths; some are short acting and some are long acting. A low starting dose is prescribed, followed by slow increases in dosage. Your doctor will determine the best dosing schedule for you. You will need to have regular blood tests to check the amount of medication in your system. After the medication is started, you may note some improvement within the first week, followed by continued lessening of symptoms over the next several weeks or months. Treatment with the medication is considered long term.

# *Missed Dose*

If you miss a dose, take it as soon as you remember. However, if it is near the time of the next dose, or the next day, skip the missed dose and resume your usual dosing schedule. *Do not double the dose in order to catch up.*

# *Side Effects*

*Side effects occur, to some degree, with all medications. They are usually not serious and do not occur in all individuals. They may sometimes occur before beneficial effects of the medication are noticed. Most side effects will decrease or disappear with time. If a side effect persists, speak to the doctor about appropriate treatment.*

You should seek immediate medical attention if you experience rash, blistering, or crusting of the skin; itching; swelling; difficulty breathing; mouth sores; lethargy; weakness; confusion; blurred vision; unusual eye movements; lack of coordination; tremor; fever or flu-like symptoms; unusual bruising; bleeding or skin blotching; yellow discoloration of the skin or yellow tinge in the eyes; nausea; vomiting; extreme loss of appetite; difficulty urinating; or dark-colored urine.

Although rare, severe liver problems may occur with anticonvulsant mood stabilizers. Contact your doctor immediately if you experience vomiting, unusual tiredness, or swelling of the face.

A rare and serious side effect of divalproex is pancreatitis. Tell your doctor immediately if you develop stomach pain, nausea, vomiting, or loss of appetite.

Common side effects that should be reported to the doctor as soon as possible include drowsiness, dizziness, dry mouth, nausea, hair loss (valproate), changes in the menstrual cycle (valproate), and weight change.

Report any other side effects not listed above to your physician.

## *Drug Interactions*

Check with the doctor or pharmacist before starting, stopping, or changing the dose of any other medicines, including over-the-counter and herbal products.

Certain antibiotics may cause carbamazepine levels to increase. Carbamazepine may make birth control pills less effective.

## *PRECAUTIONS*

- Before taking this medication, tell your doctor or pharmacist if you know you are allergic to it or if you have any other allergies.
- Take exactly as prescribed. Do not increase your dose unless instructed by your doctor. Taking too much of this medication can result in serious side effects.
- Follow your doctor's instructions regarding getting your blood levels checked.
- Do not chew or crush the tablets or capsules unless directed to do so by your doctor or pharmacist.
- Take with food or milk to prevent stomach upset.
- This medicine may cause fatigue, light-headedness, or blurred vision.

Use caution when operating machinery, driving, or performing tasks that require alertness or clear vision.

- Carbamazepine may cause increased sensitivity to sunlight.
- Do not stop taking this medication suddenly unless told to do so by your doctor. Abruptly stopping the medicine may cause your bipolar symptoms to return.
- Make sure that your doctor knows about all your medical conditions.
- Inform your doctor or pharmacist about all other medicines you are taking, including over-the-counter products.
- Avoid drinking grapefruit juice while taking carbamazepine, since it can affect the level of carbamazepine in your body.
- Do not drink alcohol while taking this medication.
- Tell your doctor if the medicine does not seem to be working or if your condition gets worse.
- Consult with your doctor if you think you might be pregnant.

- Check with your doctor before breastfeeding.
- *If you have any questions regarding this medication, do not hesitate to contact the doctor, pharmacist, or nurse.*

# PATIENT AND CAREGIVER INFORMATION ON LITHIUM

The name of your medication is ___________.

IMPORTANT NOTE: The following information is intended to supplement, not substitute for, the expertise and judgment of your physician, pharmacist, or other health care professional. It is not intended to imply that use of the drug is safe, appropriate, or effective for you. It is limited and general—in other words, it is not all-inclusive. Not all uses, side effects, precautions, or drug interactions are listed. Your doctor or pharmacist will provide you with official patient information that is more complete and detailed. Consult your health care professional before using this drug.

## *Common Brand Names*

Lithonate, Lithobid, Eskalith

## *Use*

Lithium is primarily used to treat bipolar disorder.

## *How to Use*

Lithium is available in different strengths; some varieties are short acting and some are long acting. A low starting dose is prescribed, followed by slow increases in dosage. Your doctor will determine the best dosing schedule for you. You will need to have regular blood tests to check the amount of lithium in your system. After the medication is started, you may note some improvement within the first week, followed by continued lessening of symptoms over the next several weeks or months. Treatment with the medication is considered long term.

## *Missed Dose*

If you miss a dose, take it as soon as you remember. However, if it is near the time of the next dose, or the next day, skip the missed dose and resume your usual dosing schedule. *Do not double the dose in order to catch up.*

## *Side Effects*

*Side effects occur, to some degree, with all medications. They are usually not serious and do not occur in all individuals. They may sometimes occur before beneficial effects of the medication are noticed. Most side effects will decrease or disappear with time. If a side effect persists, speak to the doctor about appropriate treatment.*

Although rare, rash, itching, swelling, or difficulty breathing sometimes occurs with lithium. Contact your doctor immediately if you experience vomiting, unusual tiredness, or swelling of the face while taking lithium.

Some side effects might mean that you have too much lithium in your system, which could be very serious. You should report the following side effects to the doctor *immediately:* clumsiness, loss of balance, feeling of intoxication, slurred speech, double vision, vomiting or diarrhea, tremors or shakiness of the hands, and change in mood or behavior.

Common side effects that should be reported to the doctor as soon as possible include difficulty concentrating, mild nausea, weight change, increased thirst and urination, and acne or skin problems.

Report any other side effects not listed above to your physician.

## *Drug Interactions*

Check with the doctor or pharmacist before starting, stopping, or changing the dose of any other medicines, including over-the-counter and herbal products.

Potentially serious drug interactions can occur with diuretic medications (water pills) and nonsteroidal anti-inflammatory medications (e.g., ibuprofen and naproxen), which can cause lithium levels to rise.

## *PRECAUTIONS*

- Before taking this medication, tell your doctor or pharmacist if you know you are allergic to it or if you have any other allergies.

- Take exactly as prescribed. Do not increase your dose unless instructed by your doctor. Taking too much lithium can result in serious side effects.
- Follow your doctor's instructions regarding getting your blood levels checked.
- Do not chew or crush the tablets or capsules unless directed to do so by your doctor or pharmacist.
- Take with food or milk to prevent stomach upset.
- Drink 8 to 12 glasses of water or other fluids every day.
- Maintain your normal diet and do not change the amount of salt in your diet unless instructed by your doctor. Limit caffeine intake.
- This medicine may cause fatigue, light-headedness, or blurred vision. Use caution when operating machinery, driving, or performing tasks that require alertness or clear vision.
- Do not stop taking your medication suddenly unless told to do so by

your doctor. Abruptly stopping the medicine may cause your bipolar symptoms to return.

- Make sure that your doctor knows about all your medical conditions.
- If you become sick with any flu-like virus or have a fever, check with your doctor to see if any changes in your lithium dose are necessary.
- Be careful not to become dehydrated when exercising, during hot weather, or any time you sweat excessively (for example, in saunas and hot tubs). Losing water and salt from your body may cause the level of lithium in your blood to increase.
- Inform your doctor or pharmacist about all other medicines you are taking, including over-the-counter products.
- Do not drink alcohol while taking this medication.
- Tell your doctor if the medicine does not seem to be working or if your condition gets worse.
- Consult with your doctor if you think you might be pregnant.
- Check with your doctor before breastfeeding.

- *If you have any questions regarding this medication, do not hesitate to contact the doctor, pharmacist, or nurse.*

# PATIENT AND CAREGIVER INFORMATION ON PSYCHOSTIMULANTS

The name of your medication is __________.

IMPORTANT NOTE: The following information is intended to supplement, not substitute for, the expertise and judgment of your physician, pharmacist, or other health care professional. It is not intended to imply that use of the drug is safe, appropriate, or effective for you. It is limited and general—in other words, it is not all-inclusive. Not all uses, side effects, precautions, or drug interactions are listed. Your doctor or pharmacist will provide you with official patient information that is more complete and detailed. Consult your health care professional before using this drug.

## *Uses*

Psychostimulants are used primarily in the treatment of attentiondeficit/hyperactivity disorder (ADHD) in children and adults. They are also approved for use in the treatment of narcolepsy.

Although they are not currently approved for this indication, psychostimulants have been found useful in the treatment of refractory depression.

The doctor may choose to use this medication for a reason not listed here. If you are not sure why this medication is being prescribed, please ask the doctor.

## *How to Use*

Take as directed, usually starting in the morning up to three times per day by mouth. Some side effects may be reduced by taking the medication with food. It is best to take it at about the same time each day. The dosage is based on your medical condition and response to therapy.

## *Missed Dose*

If you miss a dose, take it as soon as you remember. However, if it is near the time of the next dose, or the next day, skip the missed dose and resume your usual dosing schedule. *Do not double the dose in order to catch up.*

## *Side Effects*

*Side effects occur, to some degree, with all medications. They are usually not serious and do not occur in all individuals. They may sometimes occur before beneficial effects of the medication are noticed. Most side effects will decrease or disappear with time. If a side effect persists, speak to the doctor about appropriate treatment.*

Common side effects that should be reported to the doctor at the next appointment include difficulty sleeping, nervousness, excitability, loss of appetite, weight loss, increased heart rate and blood pressure, headache, nausea or heartburn, dry mouth, and dizziness.

Tell your doctor immediately if any of the following unlikely but serious side effects occurs: muscle twitches or tics; fast or irregular heartbeat; persistent throbbing headache; soreness of mouth, gums, or throat; rash; unusual bruising or bleeding; nausea and vomiting;

yellow tinge of eyes or skin; severe agitation or restlessness; *a switch in mood to an unusual state of happiness or irritability; or other fluctuations in mood.*

Report any other side effects not listed above to your physician.

## *Drug Interactions*

Because psychostimulants can change the effects of other medication or may be affected by other medication, always check with the doctor or pharmacist before taking any other drugs, including over-the-counter medication such as cold remedies. Inform all doctors and dentists who treat or examine you that you are taking a psychostimulant.

## *PRECAUTIONS*

- Before taking this medication, tell your doctor or pharmacist if you know you are allergic to it or if you have any other allergies.
- Do not increase or decrease your dose without consulting your doctor.

- *If you have any questions regarding this medication, do not hesitate to contact the doctor, pharmacist, or nurse.*

# PATIENT AND CAREGIVER INFORMATION ON ANTIPSYCHOTICS

The name of your medication is ___________.

IMPORTANT NOTE: The following information is intended to supplement, not substitute for, the expertise and judgment of your physician, pharmacist, or other health care professional. It is not intended to imply that use of the drug is safe, appropriate, or effective for you. It is limited and general—in other words, it is not all-inclusive. Not all uses, side effects, precautions, or drug interactions are listed. Your doctor or pharmacist will provide you with official patient information that is more complete and detailed. Consult your health care professional before using this drug.

## *Uses*

Antipsychotics are used to treat certain mental and mood conditions, such as schizophrenia and bipolar mania. They work by helping to restore the balance of certain natural chemicals in the brain (neurotransmitters). Some of the benefits of continued use include reduced nervousness, better concentration, and reduced episodes of confusion.

## *How to Use*

Take as directed, usually once a day by mouth with or without food. Stand up slowly, especially when starting this medication, to avoid dizziness. The dosage is based on your medical condition and response to therapy. Use this medication regularly in order to get the most benefit from it. Remember to use it at the same time each day.

## *Missed Dose*

If you miss a dose, take it as soon as you remember. However, if it is near the time of the next dose, or the next day, skip the missed dose and resume your usual dosing schedule. *Do not double the dose in order to catch up.*

# *Side Effects*

*Side effects occur, to some degree, with all medications. They are usually not serious and do not occur in all individuals. They may sometimes occur before beneficial effects of the medication are noticed. Most side effects will decrease or disappear with time. If a side effect persists, speak to the doctor about appropriate treatment.*

Common side effects that should be reported to the doctor at the next appointment include dizziness, stomach pain, dry mouth, constipation, weight gain, and drowsiness. If any of these effects persists or worsens, notify your doctor or pharmacist promptly.

To minimize dizziness or fainting, stand up slowly when rising from a seated or lying position, especially when you first start using this medication.

Tell your doctor immediately if any of the following unlikely but serious side effects occurs: fast heartbeat, ankle or leg swelling, agitation, confusion, restlessness, weakness, difficulty speaking, numbness or tingling of hands or feet, trouble walking (abnormal gait), painful menstrual periods, pink urine, tremor, muscle spasm or rigidity, chest pain, yellowing of the eyes or skin, one-sided weakness, sudden vision changes or other eye problems, headache, painful urination, seizures, or difficulty swallowing.

This drug infrequently causes blood sugar levels to rise, which can cause or worsen diabetes. High blood sugar can, in rare cases, cause serious (sometimes fatal) conditions such as diabetic coma. Tell your doctor immediately if you develop symptoms of high blood sugar, such as unusual increased thirst and urination. If you already have diabetes, be sure to check your blood sugar levels regularly.

This medication may also cause significant weight gain and a rise in your blood cholesterol (or triglyceride) levels. These effects, along with diabetes, may increase your risk of heart disease. Discuss the risks and benefits of treatment with your doctor.

This medication can in rare cases cause a serious condition called neuroleptic malignant syndrome (NMS). Tell your doctor immediately if you develop any of the following symptoms: fever, muscle stiffness, severe confusion, sweating, or fast or irregular heartbeat.

In rare cases, antipsychotics cause a condition known as tardive dyskinesia. In some cases, this condition may be permanent. Tell your doctor immediately if you develop any unusual or uncontrolled movements (especially of the face or tongue).

Report any other side effects not listed above to your physician.

## *Drug Interactions*

Before using this medication, tell your doctor or pharmacist about all prescription medications and over-the-counter or herbal products you are using, especially carbamazepine (Tegretol, Equetro), fluvoxamine (Luvox), omeprazole (Prilosec), rifampin (Rifadin), drugs for high blood pressure, and drugs for Parkinson's disease.

Report drugs that cause drowsiness as well, because this effect will be increased by taking them in combination with this medication.

Do not start or stop any medicine without doctor or pharmacist approval.

## *PRECAUTIONS*

- Before taking this medication, tell your doctor or pharmacist if you know you are allergic to it or if you have any other allergies.
- Do not increase or decrease your dose without consulting your doctor.
- This drug may make you dizzy or drowsy; use caution when engaging in activities requiring alertness, such as riding a bike, driving, or using machinery.
- Avoid alcoholic beverages.
- Avoid excessive amounts of caffeine.
- This medication can make you prone to heat stroke. Avoid activities that might cause you to overheat (such as doing strenuous work, exercising in hot weather, and using hot tubs).
- Do not share this medication with others.
- Laboratory and/or medical tests (such as fasting blood sugar, weight, blood pressure, blood

cholesterol/triglyceride levels, and liver function tests) should be performed periodically to monitor your progress and check for side effects. Consult your doctor for more details.

- Go for regular eye exams as part of your regular health care regimen, and to check for any unlikely, but possible, eye problems.
- *If you have any questions regarding this medication, do not hesitate to contact the doctor, pharmacist, or nurse.*

# PATIENT AND CAREGIVER INFORMATION ON SLEEP MEDICATIONS

The name of your medication is __________.

IMPORTANT NOTE: The following information is intended to supplement, not substitute for, the expertise and judgment of your physician, pharmacist, or other health care professional. It is not intended to imply that use of the drug is safe, appropriate, or effective for you. It is limited and general—in other words, it is not all-inclusive. Not all uses, side effects, precautions, or drug interactions are listed. Your doctor or pharmacist will provide you with official patient information that is more complete and detailed. Consult your health care professional before using this drug.

## *Uses*

Medications from different classes are used to treat sleep disorders such as insomnia, nightmares, and other disorders. These classes include sedative-hypnotics (Ambien, Lunesta, Restoril), certain antidepressants (Trazodone, Remeron, Doxepin), antihistamines (Vistaril, Benadryl), and others. Each class works differently, but they share the primary effect of inducing sedation. Some of the benefits of use include increased quality and quantity of sleep, reduced daytime fatigue, and elimination of or reduction in nightmares.

## *How to Use*

Take as directed, usually once a day by mouth approximately 30 to 60 minutes prior to bedtime. The dosage is based on your medical condition, response to therapy, age, and possibly weight. Use this medication as prescribed by your health care provider in order to get the most benefit from it. It is important to give yourself at least 8 hours between the time you take the medication and your scheduled time to wake up. Sleep medications are often used on an "as needed" basis and not taken every day. Consult your health care provider if you are unsure how to take the medication. It is important that you are ready for bed prior to taking the medication.

## *Side Effects*

*Side effects occur, to some degree, with all medications. They are usually not serious and do not occur in all individuals. They may sometimes occur before beneficial effects of the medication are noticed. Most side effects will decrease or disappear with time. If a side effect persists, speak to your health care provider about appropriate treatment.*

Common side effects that should be reported to the doctor at the next appointment include dizziness, dry mouth, constipation, vivid dreams or nightmares, or weight gain. You should notify your doctor or pharmacist promptly if you experience daytime drowsiness, difficulty waking up, memory lapses, or suicidal thinking.

To minimize dizziness or fainting, stand up slowly when rising from a seated or lying position, especially when you first start using this medication.

Tell your doctor immediately if any of the following unlikely but serious side effects occurs: fast or irregular heartbeat, ankle or leg swelling, agitation, confusion, restlessness, weakness, difficulty speaking, numbness or tingling of hands or feet, trouble walking (abnormal gait), painful menstrual periods, erections lasting longer than four hours, pink urine, tremor, muscle spasm or rigidity, chest pain, yellowing of the eyes or skin, one-sided weakness, sudden vision changes or other eye problems, headache, painful urination, seizures, or difficulty swallowing.

Report any other side effects not listed above to your physician.

## *Drug Interactions*

Before using this medication, tell your doctor or pharmacist about all prescription medications and over-the-counter or herbal products you are using, especially antidepressants, antihistamines, sedatives (e.g., benzodiazepines), and other medications with the known side effect of drowsiness.

Do not start or stop any medicine without doctor or pharmacist approval.

## *PRECAUTIONS*

- Before taking this medication, tell your doctor or pharmacist if you know you are allergic to it or if you have any other allergies.
- Do not increase or decrease your dose without consulting your doctor.
- Do not take more frequently than as prescribed.
- This drug may make you dizzy or drowsy; do not engage in activities requiring alertness, such as riding a bike, driving, or using machinery.
- Avoid alcoholic beverages.
- Do not take with over-the-counter sleep aids.
- Do not share this medication with others.
- *If you have any questions regarding this medication, do not hesitate to contact the doctor, pharmacist, or nurse.*

# References

American Diabetes Association, the American Psychiatric Association, & the American Association of Clinical Endocrinologists. (2004). Consensus development conference on antipsychotic drugs and obesity and diabetes. *Journal of Clinical Psychiatry, 65,* 267–272.

American Psychiatric Association (1980). *Diagnostic and Statistical Manual of Mental Disorders, Third Edition (DSM-III).* Washington, DC: American Psychiatric Association Publishing.

American Psychiatric Association. (1987). *Diagnostic and Statistical Manual of Mental Disorders (DSM-III-R)* (3rd ed., Rev. ed.). Washington, DC: American Psychiatric Association Publishing.

American Psychiatric Association. (2000). *Diagnostic and Statistical Manual of Mental Disorders (DSM-IV-TR)* (4th ed., Text revision). Washington, DC:

American Psychiatric Association Publishing.

American Psychiatric Association. (2013). *Diagnostic and Statistical Manual of Mental Disorders (DSM-V)* (5th ed.). Washington, DC: American Psychiatric Association Publishing.

Amsterdam, J.D., Li, Y., Soeller, I., Rockwell, K., Mao, J.J., & Shults, J. (2009). A randomized, double-blind, placebo controlled trial of oral *Matricaria recutita* (chamomile) extract treatment for generalized anxiety disorder. *Journal of Clinical Psychopharmacology, 29*(4), 378–382.

Asperger, H. (1991). Die "Autistischen Psychopathen" im Kindesalter. In *Autism and Asperger Syndrome,* pp.37–92. (U. Frith, Trans.). Cambridge, England: Cambridge University Press. (Original work published 1944).

Aursnes, I., I.F. Tvete, J. Gaasemyr, & B. Natvig. (2005). Suicide attempts in clinical trials with paroxetine randomised against placebo. *BMC Medicine* 3:14. doi: 10/1186/1741-701 5-3-14

Barkley, R.A. (2000). *Taking Charge of ADHD: The Complete, Authoritative Guide for Parents (Revised Edition).* New York: Guilford Press.

Barnhart, W.J., Makela, E.H., & Latocha, M.J. (2004). SSRI-induced apathy syndrome: A clinical review. *Journal of Psychiatric Practice, 10*(3), 196–199.

Bender, K.J. (Ed.). (1993). Narcotic antagonist for alcoholism. *Psychotropics, 13,* 6–8.

Berger, S., Kugler, J.D., Thomas, J.A., & Friedberg, D.Z. (2004). Sudden cardiac death in children and adolescents: Introduction and overview. *Pediatric Clinics of North America, 51*(5), 1201–1209.

Biederman, J., Wilens, T., Mick, E., Spencer, T., & Faraone, S.V. (1999). Pharmacotherapy for attention-deficit/hyperactivity disorder reduces risk for substance abuse disorder. *Pediatrics, 104*(2), e20.

Biederman, J., Hirshfeld-Becker, D.R., Rosenbaum, J.F., Hérot, C., Friedman, D., Snidman, N., et al. (2001). Further evidence of association between behavioral inhibition and social anxiety in children. *American Journal of Psychiatry, 158,* 1673–1679.

Biederman, J., Mick, E., Faraone, S.V., Spencer, T., Wilens, T.E., & Wozniak, J. (2003). Current concepts in the validity, diagnosis, and treatment of paediatric bipolar disorder. *International Journal of Neuropsychopharmacology, 6,* 293–300.

Biederman, J., Wilens, T., Mick, E., Spencer, T., & Faraone, S.V. (1999). Pharmacotherapy for attention-deficit/hyperactivity disorder reduces risk for substance abuse disorder. *Pediatrics, 104*(2), e20.

Birmaher, B. (2013). "Longitudinal trajectory of childhood bipolar disorder." Presented at the 60th Annual Meeting of the American Academy of Child and Adolescent Psychiatry, Buena Vista, FL, October 22–27.

Birmaher, B., Kennah, H., Brent, D., Ehmann, M., Bridge, J., & Axelson, D. (2002). Is bipolar disorder specifically associated with panic disorder in youths? *Journal of Clinical Psychiatry, 63*(5), 414–419.

Bloch, M.H., & Hannestad, J. (2012). Omega-3 fatty acids for the treatment of depression: Systematic review and meta-analysis. *Molecular Psychiatry, 17*(12), 1272–1282.

Bloch, M.H., Landeros-Weisenberger, A., Kelmendi, B., Cohen, D.J., & Price, L.H. (2006). A systematic review: Antipsychotic augmentation with treatment refractory obsessive-compulsive disorder. *Molecular Psychiatry, 11*(7), 622–632.

Bowes, M. (2001). OCD: Will immunotherapy succeed where other approaches have failed? *Neuropsychiatry Reviews, 2,* 1–25.

Brangham, W. (2014). Is pot getting more potent? *PBS NewsHour.* Retrieved from http://www.pbs.org/newshour/updates/pot-getting-potent/

Brent, D. (2013). Depression in youth is tough to treat and requires persistence and creativity. Presented at the 60th Annual Meeting of the American Academy of Child and Adolescent Psychiatry annual meeting, Buena Vista, FL, October 22–27. Also noted in *Bipolar Network News, 17*(6), 1–2.

Brodkin, E.S., McDougle, C.J., Naylor, S.T., et al. (1997). Clomipramine in adults with pervasive developmental disorder: A prospective open-label investigation. *Journal of Child and Adolescent Psychopharmacology,* 7(2), 109–121.

Brotman, A. (1992). *Practical Reviews in Psychiatry.* Birmingham, AL: Educational Reviews [audiotape].

Brown University. (2004). Experts, parents weigh in at FDA's public hearing on SSRI safety. *Child and Adolescent Psychopharmacology Update, 6*(3), 1–3.

Calhoun, S.L., Fernandez-Mendoza, J., Vgontzas, A.N., Liao, D., & Bixler, E.O. (2014). Prevalence of insomnia symptoms in a general population sample of young children and preadolescents: Gender effects. *Sleep Medicine, 15*(1), 91–95.

Campaign for a Commercial-Free Childhood (2014). https://commercialfreechildhood.org

Campbell, M., Anderson, L.T., Small, A.M., Adams, P., Gonzalez, N.M., & Ernst, M. (1993). Naltrexone in autistic children: Behavioral symptoms and attentional learning. *Journal of the American Academy of Child and Adolescent Psychiatry, 32,* 1283–1291.

Carlat, D. (2006). Bipolar disorder in children: Is the diagnosis valid? *The Carlat Psychiatry Report, 4*(8), 1–2.

Carlson, G.A., Bromet, E.J., & Sievers, S. (2000). Phenomenology and outcome of subjects with early-and adult-onset psychotic mania. *American Journal of Psychiatry, 157*(2), 213–219.

Carlson, G.A., Jensen, P.S., Findling, R.L., Meyer, R.E., Calabrese, J., DelBello, M.P., et al. (2003). Methodological issues and controversies in clinical trials with child and adolescent patients with bipolar disorder: Report of a consensus conference. *Journal of Child and Adolescent Psychopharmacology, 13*(1), 13–27.

Center on Addiction. (2011a) (June). National study reveals: Teen substance use: America's #1 public health problem. Retrieved from https://www.centeronaddiction.org/newsroom/press-releases/national-study-reveals-teen-substance-use-america%E2%80%99s-1-public-health-problem

Center on Addiction. (2011b) (August 24). 2011 national teen survey finds: Teens regularly using social networking sites likelier to smoke, drink, use drugs. Retrieved from https://www.centeronaddiction.org/newsroom/press-releases/2011-national-teen-survey-finds

Chang, S.J. & Chae, K.Y. (2010). Obstructive sleep apnea syndrome in children: Epidemiology, pathophysiology, diagnosis, and sequelae. *Korean Journal of Pediatrics, 53*(10), 863–871.

Cohen, J.A., Mannarino, A.P., & Deblinger, E. (2017). *Treating Trauma and Traumatic Grief in Children and Adolescents, Second Edition.* New York: The Guilford Press.

Coletti, D.J., Leigh, E., Gallelli, K.A., & Kafantaris, V. (2005). Patterns of adherence to treatment in adolescents with bipolar disorder. *Journal of Child and Adolescent Psychopharmacology, 15,* 913–917.

Conners, K. (2008). *Conners 3rd Edition.* Multi-Health Systems, Inc.

Connor, D.F., Grasso, D.J., Slivinsky, M.D., Pearson, G.S., & Banga, A.

(2013). An open-label study of guanfacine extended release for traumatic stress related symptoms in children and adolescents. *Journal of Child and Adolescent Psychopharmacology, 23*(4), 244–251.

Cook, E.H., Wagner, K.D., March, J.S., Biederman, J., Landau, P., Wolkow, R., et al. (2001). Long-term sertraline treatment of children and adolescents with obsessive-compulsive disorder. *Journal of Child and Adolescent Psychopharmacology, 40,* 1175–1181.

Costello, E.J., Pine, D.S., Hammen, C., March, J.S., Plotsky, P.M., Weissman, M.M., et al. (2002). Development and natural history of mood disorders. *Biological Psychiatry, 52,* 529–542.

Coyle, J.T., Pine, D.S., Charney, D.S., Lewis, L., Nemeroff, C.F., Carlson, G.A., et al. (2003). Depression and bipolar support alliance consensus statement on the unmet needs in diagnosis and treatment of mood disorders in children and adolescents. *Journal of the*

*American Academy of Child and Adolescent Psychiatry, 42,* 1494–1503.

Di Forti, M., Morgan, C., Dazzan P., Pariante, C., Mondelli V., Marques T.R., et al. (2009) High-potency cannabis and the risk of psychosis. *British Journal of Psychiatry, 195*(6): 488-491.

DelBello, M. (2013). Omega-3 fatty acids promising for at-risk children with depression. *Bipolar Network News, 17*(6), 2.

Doshi, J.A., Hodgkins, P., Kahle, J., Sikirica, V., Cangelosi, M.J., Setyawan, J., et al. (2012). Economic impact of childhood and adult attention-deficit/hyperactivity disorder in the United States. *Journal of the American Academy of Child and Adolescent Psychiatry, 51*(10), 990–1102.

Eddy, C.M., Rickards, H.E., & Cavanna, A.E. (2011). Treatment strategies for tics in Tourette syndrome. *Therapeutic Advances in Neurological Disorders, 4*(1), 25–45.

Emslie, G.J., & Mayes, T.C. (2001). Mood disorders in children and adolescents: Psychopharmacological treatment. *Biological Psychiatry, 49,* 1082–1090.

Falkowitz, S., Akbar, N., & Greenhill, L. (2017). Attention-deficit/hyperactivity disorder. In M. McVoy and R.L. Findling (Eds.). *Clinical Manual of Child and Adolescent Psychopharmacology, Third Edition,* pp.35–107. Arlington, VA: American Psychiatric Association Publishing.

Faraone, S.V., Spencer, T., Aleardi, M., Pagano, C., & Biederman, J. (2004). Meta-analysis of the efficacy of methylphenidate for treating adult attention-deficit/hyperactivity disorder. *Journal of Clinical Psychopharmacology, 24*(1), 24–29.

Findling, R.L., McNamara, N.K., Gracious, B.L., Youngstrom, E.A., Stansbrey, R.J., Reed, M.D., et al. (2003). Combination lithium and divalproex sodium in pediatric bipolarity. *Journal of the American*

*Academy of Child and Adolescent Psychiatry, 42,* 895–901.

Gangwisch, J.E., Babiss, L.A., Malaspina, D., Turner, J.B., Zammit, G.K., Posner, K. (2010). Earlier parental set bedtimes as a protective factor against depression and suicidal ideation. *Sleep, 33*(1), 97–106.

Geller, B., Craney, J.L., Bolhofner, K., Nickelsburg, M.J., Williams, M., & Zimerman, B. (2002). Two-year prospective follow-up of children with a prepubertal and early adolescent bipolar disorder phenotype. *American Journal of Psychiatry, 159,* 927–933.

Geller, B., & DelBello, M.P. (Eds.). (2003). *Bipolar Disorder in Childhood and Early Adolescence.* New York: Guilford Press.

Geller, B., Luby, J.L., Joshi, P., Wagner, K.D., Emslie, G., Walkup, J.T., et al. (2012). A randomized controlled trial of risperidone, lithium, or divalproex sodium for initial treatment of bipolar I disorder, manic or mixed phase, in children and adolescents. *Archives of General Psychiatry, 69*(5), 515–528.

Geller, B., Sun, K., Zimerman, B., Luby, J., Frazier, J., & Williams, M. (1995). Complex and rapid-cycling in bipolar children and adolescents: A preliminary study. *Journal of Affective Disorders, 34,* 259–268.

Gibbons, R.D., Brown, C.H., Hur, K., Davis, J.M., & Mann, J.J. (2012). Suicidal thoughts and behavior with antidepressant treatment: Re-analysis of the randomized placebo-controlled studies of fluoxetine and venlafaxine. *Archives of General Psychiatry, 69*(6), 580–587.

Gillman, P.K. (2007). Tricyclic antidepressant pharmacology and therapeutic drug interactions updated. *British Journal of Pharmacology, 151*(6), 737–748.

Glass, R.M. (2004). Treatment of adolescents with major depression: Contributions of a major trial. *Journal of the American Medical Association, 292*(7), 861–863.

Greenhill, L.L., Abikoff, H.B., Arnold, L.E., Cantwell, D.P., Conners, C.K., Elliott, G., et al. (1996). Medication treatment strategies in the MTA Study: Relevance to clinicians and researchers. *Journal of the American Academy of Child and Adolescent Psychiatry, 35,* 1304–1313.

Groenman, A.P., Oosterlann, J., Rommelse, N.N., Franke, B., Hoekstra, P.J., Hartman, C.A., et al. (2013). Stimulant treatment for attention-deficit hyperactivity disorder and risk of developing substance use disorder. *British Journal of Psychiatry,* 203(2)112–119.

Heller, T. (1908). Dementia infantilis. *Zeitschrift fu□r die Erforschung und Behandlung des jugendlichen Schwachsinns, 2,* 141–165.

Heo, Y.A. & Duggan, S.T. (2017). Lisdexamfetamine: A review in binge eating disorder. *CNS Drugs, 31*(11), 1015–1022.

Ho, F.Y., Chan, C.S., & Tang, K.N. (2016). Cognitive-behavioral therapy for sleep disturbances in treating posttraumatic stress disorder symptoms: A meta-analysis of randomized clinical trials. *Clinical Psychology Review, 43,* 90–102.

Jacobson, R. (2014, March 1). Should children take antipsychotic drugs? *Scientific American Mind, 25*(2), 13.

Jureidini, J., Doecke, C.J., Mansfield, P.R., Haby, M.M., Menkes, D.B., & Tonkin, A.L. (2004). Efficacy and safety of antidepressants for children and adolescents. *British Medical Journal, 328,* 879-883.

Kagan, J. (1998). *Galen's Prophecy: Temperament in Human Nature.* New York: Basic Books.

Kanner, L. (1943). Autistic disturbances of affective contact. *Nervous Child, 2,* 217–250.

Keck, P., McElroy, S., Strakowski, S., West, S., Sax, K., Hawkins, J., et al. (1998). 12-month outcome of patients with bipolar disorder following hospitalization for a manic or mixed episode. *American Journal of Psychiatry, 155,* 646–652.

Kent, J.M., Kushner, S., Ning, X., Karcher, K., Ness, S., Aman, M., et al. (2013). Risperidone dosing in children and adolescents with autistic disorder: A double-blind, placebo-controlled study. *Journal of Autism and Development Disorders, 43*(8), 1773–1783.

Kerr, A.M., Armstrong, D.D., Prescott, R.J., Doyle, D., & Kearney, D.L. (1997). Rett syndrome: Analysis of death in the British survey. *European Child and Adolescent Psychiatry 6*(Suppl. 1), 71–74.

Kolmen, B.K., Feldman, H.M., Handen, B.L., & Janosky, J.E. (1995). Naltrexone in young autistic children: A double-blind, placebo-controlled crossover study. *Journal of the*

*American Academy of Child and Adolescent Psychiatry, 34,* 223–231.

Kowatch, R.A., Suppes, T., Carmody, T.J., Bucci, J.P., Hume, J.H., Kromelis, M., & Child Psychiatric Workgroup on Bipolar Disorder. (2000). Effect size of lithium, divalproex sodium, and carbamazepine in children and adolescents with bipolar disorder. *Journal of the American Academy of Child and Adolescent Psychiatry, 39,* 713–720.

Kowatch, R.A., Fristad, M., Birmaher, B., Wagner, K., Findling, R., & Hellander, M. (2005). Treatment guidelines for children and adolescents with bipolar disorder. *Journal of the American Academy of Child and Adolescent Psychiatry, 44,* 213–235.

Kuczenski, R., & Segal, D.S. (2002). Exposure of adolescent rats to oral methylphenidate: Preferential effects on extracellular norepinephrine and absence of sensitization and cross-sensitization to methamphetamine.

*Journal of Neuroscience, 22,* 7 264–7271.

Lewinsohn, P.M., Klein, D.N., & Seeley, J.R. (1995). Bipolar disorders in a community sample of older adolescents: Prevalence, phenomenology, comorbidity, and course. *Journal of the American Academy of Child and Adolescent Psychiatry, 34*(4), 454–463.

Lewinsohn, P.M., Klein, D.N., & Seeley, J.R. (2000). Bipolar disorder during adolescence and young adulthood in a community sample. *Bipolar Disorder, 2*(3 Pt 2), 281–293.

Li, S.X.,, Yu, M.W., Lam, S.P., Zhang, J., Li, A.M., Lai, K.Y., & Wing, Y.K. (2011). Frequent nightmares in children: Familial aggregation and associations with parent-reported behavioral and mood problems. *Sleep, 34*(4), 487–493.

Liebenluft, E., Charney, D.S., Towbin, K.E., Bhangoo, R.K., & Pine, D.S. (2003). Defining clinical phenotypes of juvenile mania. *American Journal of Psychiatry, 160,* 430–437.

Linde, K., Berner, M.M., & Kriston, L. (2008). St. John's wort for major depression. *Cochrane Database of Systematic Reviews,* 2008(4), CD000448.

Locher, C., Koechlin, H., Zion, S.R., Werner, C., Pine, D.S., Kirsch, et al. (2017). Efficacy and safety of selective serotonin reuptake inhibitors, serotonin-norepinephrine reuptake inhibitors, and placebo for common psychiatric disorders among children and adolescents: A Systematic Review and Meta-analysis. *JAMA Psychiatry, 74*(10), 1011–1020.

Luby, E.D., Marrazzi, M.A., & Kinzie, J. (1987). Treatment of chronic anorexia nervosa with opiate blockade. *Journal of Clinical Psychopharmacology, 7,* 52–53.

Luby, J.L., Heffelfinger, A.K., Mrakosky, C., Hessler, M.J., Brown, K.M., & Hildebrand, T. (2002). Preschool major depressive disorder: Preliminary validation for developmentally modified *DSM-IV* criteria. *Journal of the American Academy of Child and Adolescent Psychiatry, 41*(8), 928–937.

Lynch, M., Rabin, R.A., & George, T.P. (2012). The cannabis-psychosis link. *Psychiatric Times.* Retrieved from http://www.psychiatrictimes.com/schizophrenia/cannabis-psychosis-link

Mahler, J. (2004, November 21). The antidepressant dilemma. *New York Times Magazine,* p.59.

Mannuzza, S., Klein, R.G., & Moulton, J.L., III. (2003). Does stimulant treatment place children at risk for adult substance abuse? A controlled, prospective follow-up study. *Journal of Child and Adolescent Psychopharmacology, 13*(3), 273–282.

March, J.S., Franklin, M., Nelson, A., & Foa, E. (2001). Cognitivebehavioral psychotherapy for pediatric obsessive-compulsive disorder. *Journal of Clinical Child Psychology, 30,* 8–18.

March, J., Silva, J., Petrycki, S., Curry, J., Wells, K., Fairbank, J., et al. (2004). Fluoxetine, cognitive-behavioral therapy and their combination for adolescents with depression: Treatment for Adolescents With Depression Study (TADS) randomized controlled trial. *Journal of the American Medical Association, 292,* 807–820.

Masi, G., Perugi, G., Toni, C., Millepiedi, S., Mucci, M., Bertini, N., & Akiskal, H.S. (2004). Obsessive-compulsive bipolar comorbidity: Focus on children and adolescents. *Journal of Affective Disorders, 78*(3), 175–183.

McDougle, C.J., Holmes, J.P., Carlson, D.C., Pelton, G.H., Cohen, D.J., & Price, L.H. (1998). A double-blind, placebo-controlled study of risperidone in adults with autistic disorder and other pervasive developmental disorders. *Archives of General Psychiatry, 55*(7), 633–641.

Merikangas, K.R., He, J.P., Burstein, M., Swanson, S.A., Avenevoli, S., Cui, L., et al. (2010). Lifetime prevalence of mental disorders in U.S. adolescents: Results from the National Comorbidity Survey Replication—Adolescent Supplement (NCS-A). *Journal of American Academy of Child and Adolescent Psychiatry, 49*(10), 980–989.

Moreno, C., Laje, G., Blanco, C., Jiang, H., Schmidt, A.B., & Olfson, M. (2007). National trends in the outpatient diagnosis and treatment of bipolar disorder in youth. *Archives of General Psychiatry, 64*(9), 1032–1039.

The MTA Cooperative Group. (1999). A 14-month randomized clinical trial of treatment strategies for attention-deficit/hyperactivity disorder. *Archives of General Psychiatry, 56*(12), 1073–1086.

Munetz, M.R., Benjamin, S. (1988). How to examine patients using the Abnormal Involuntary Movement Scale. *Hospital and Community Psychiatry, 39*(11), 1172–1177.

National Institute of Mental Health. Systematic Treatment Enhancement

Program for Bipolar Disorder (STEP-BD). (ND). Retrieved from https://www.nimh.nih.gov/funding/clinical-research/practical/step-bd/index.shtml

National Institutes of Health. (2014, May). Melatonin. *Medline Plus.* Retrieved from https://www.nccih.nih.gov/health/melatonin-what-you-need-to-know

Nobile, M., Cataldo, G.M., Marino, C., & Molteni, M. (2003). Diagnosis and treatment of dysthymia in children and adolescents. *CNS Drugs, 17*(13), 927–946.

Nottelmann E., Biederman, J., Birmaher, B., Carlson, G., Chang, K.D., Frenton W.S., et al. (2000). Roundtable on prepubertal bipolar disorder. *Journal of the American Academy of Child and Adolescent Psychiatry, 40*(8), 871–878.

Ollendick, T.H., Öst, L.-G., Reuterskiöld, L., & Costa, N. (2010). Comorbidity in youth with specific phobias: Impact of comorbidity on treatment outcome and the impact of treatment on comorbid disorders. *Behaviour Research and Therapy, 48*(9), 827–831.

Palumbo, M.L., Keary, C.J., & McDougle, C.J. (2017). Autism spectrum disorder. In M. McVoy & R.L. Findling (eds.)., *Clinical Manual of Child and Adolescent Psychopharmacology, Third Edition,* pp.307–361. Arlington, VA: American Psychiatric Association.

Papolos, D., & Papolos, J. (2007). *The Bipolar Child: The Definitive and Reassuring Guide to Childhood's Most Misunderstood Disorder, Third Edition.* New York: Broadway Books.

Pappadopulos, E., Jensen, P.S., Chait, A.R., Arnold, L.E., Swanson, J.M., Greenhilll, L.L., et al. (2009). Medication adherence in the MTA: Saliva methylphenidate samples versus parent report and mediating effect of concomitant behavioral treatment. *Journal of the American Academy of Child and Adolescent Psychiatry, 48*(5), 501–510.

Pediatric OCD Treatment Study (POTS) Team. (2004). Cognitive-behavior therapy, sertraline, and their combination for children and adolescents with obsessive-compulsive disorder: The Pediatric OCD Treatment Study (POTS) randomized controlled trial. *Journal of the American Medical Association, 292*(16), 1969–1976.

Picchietti, M.A. & Picchietti, D.L. (2008). Restless legs and periodic limb movement disorder in children and adolescents. *Seminars in Pediatric Neurology, 15*(2), 91–99.

Pliszka, S., Greenhill, L.L., Crismon, M.L., Sedillo, A., Carlson, C., Conners, C.K., et al. (2000). The Texas Children's Medication Algorithm Project: Report of the Texas Consensus Conference Panel on Medication Treatment of Childhood Attention Deficit/Hyperactivity Disorder: Part I. Attention-deficit/hyperactivity disorder. *Journal of the American Academy of Child and Adolescent Psychiatry, 39*(7), 908–927.

Popper, C. (2004). Bipolar disorder in children and adolescents. *Audio Digest Psychiatry, 33*(2).

Post, R. (2013). Omega-3 fatty acids promising for at-risk kids with depression. *Bipolar Network News.* Retrieved from https://bipolarnews.org/?m=201311

Preti, A., Melis, M., Siddi, S., Vellante, M., Doneddu, G., & Fadda, R. (2014). Oxytocin and autism: A systematic review of randomized controlled trials. *Journal of Child and Adolescent Psychopharmacology, 24*(2), 54–68.

Purdon, S.E., Lit, W., Labelle, A., & Jones, B.D. (1994). Risperidone in the treatment of pervasive developmental disorder. *Canadian Journal of Psychiatry, 39,* 400–405.

Qin, B., Zhang, Y., Zhou, X., Cheng, P., Liu, Y., Chen, J., et al. (2014). Selective serotonin reuptake inhibitors versus tricyclic antidepressants in young patients: A meta-analysis of efficacy and acceptability. *Clinical Therapeutics, 36*(7), 1087–1095.

Research Unit on Pediatric Psychopharmacology Anxiety Study Group. (2001). Fluvoxamine for the treatment of anxiety disorders in children and adolescents. *New England Journal of Medicine, 344,* 1279–1285.

Rett, A. (1977). *Uber ein zerebral-atrophisches Syndrom bei Hyperammoniamie.* [A cerebral atrophy associated with hyperammonaemia.] In P.J. Vinken & G.W. Bruyn (Eds.), *Handbook of Clinical Neurology.* Amsterdam, North-Holland. (Original work published 1966).

Robertson, M.M., & Stern, J.S. (1997). The Gilles de la Tourette syndrome. *Critical Reviews in Neurobiology, 11,* 1–19.

Sachs, G.S., Baldassano, C.F., Truman, C.J., & Guille, C. (2000). Comorbidity of attention deficit hyperactivity disorder with early-and late-onset bipolar disorder. *American Journal of Psychiatry, 157,* 466–468.

Safer, D.J., & Krager, J.M. (1992). Effect of a media blitz and a threatened lawsuit on stimulant treatment. *Journal of the American Medical Association, 268,* 1004–1007.

Schwartz, C.E., Snidman, N., & Kagan, J. (1999). Adolescent social anxiety as an outcome of inhibited temperament in childhood. *Journal of the American Academy of Child and Adolescent Psychiatry, 38,* 1008–1015.

Shaw, K., Turner, J., & Del Mar, C. (2002). Tryptophan and 5-hydroxytryptophan for depression. *Cochrane Database of Systemic Reviews, 1,* CD003198.

Simard, V. & Nielsen, T.A. (2009). Adaptation of imagery rehearsal therapy for nightmares in children: A brief report. *Psychotherapy: Theory, Research, Practice, Training, 46*(4), 492–497.

Simard, V., Nielsen, T.A., Tremblay, R.E., Boivin, M., & Montplaisir, J.Y. (2008). Longitudinal study of bad dreams in preschool-aged children: Prevalence, demographic correlates, risk and protective factors. *Sleep, 31*(1), 62–70.

Sinclair, L. (2013, April 19). ADHD meds may not cut risk for drug abuse in teens. *Psychiatric News.* Retrieved from https://psychnews.psychiatryonline.org/doi/full/10.1176/appi.pn.2013.4a6

Smoller, J.W. & Finn, C.T. (2003). Family, twin, and adoption studies of bipolar disorder. *American Journal of Medical Genetics. Part C, Seminars in Medical Genetics, 123C*(1), 48–58.

Snider, L.A., & Swedo, S.E. (2004). PANDAS: Current status and directions for research. *Molecular Psychiatry, 10,* 900–907.

St.-Onge, M., Mercier, P., & De Koninck, J. (2009). Imagery rehearsal therapy for frequent nightmares in children. *Behavioral Sleep Medicine, 7*(2), 81–98.

Stahl, S.M. (2013). *Stahl's Essential Psychopharmacology: Neuroscientific Basis and Practical Applications, Fourth Edition.* New York: Cambridge University Press.

Stahl, S.M. (2018). *Stahl's Essential Psychopharmacology Prescriber's Guide: Children and Adolescents, First Edition.* New York: Cambridge University Press.

Stern, E., Silbersweig, D.A., Chee, K., Holmes, A., Robertson, M.M., Trimble, M., et al. (2000). A functional neuroanatomy of tics in Tourette syndrome. *Archives of General Psychiatry, 57,* 741–748.

Taylor, M.J., Carney, S.M., Geddes, J., & Goodwin, G. (2003). Folate for depressive disorders. *Cochrane Database of Systemic Reviews 2, CD003390.*

Thomsen, P.H., Ebbesen, C., & Persson, C. (2001). Long-term experience with citalopram in the treatment of adolescent OCD. *Journal of the*

*American Academy of Child and Adolescent Psychiatry, 40,* 895–902.

Tsuang, M.T., & Faraone, S.V. (1990.) *The Genetics of Mood Disorders.* Baltimore: Johns Hopkins University Press.

Vetter, V.L., Elia, J., Erickson, C., Berger, S., Blum, N., Uzark, K., et al. American Heart Association Council on Cardiovascular Nursing. (2008). Cardiovascular monitoring of children and adolescents with heart disease receiving medications for attention deficit/hyperactivity disorder [corrected]: A scientific statement from the American Heart Association Council on Cardiovascular Disease in the Young Congenital Cardiac Defects Committee and the Council on Cardiovascular Nursing. *Circulation, 117*(18), 2407–2423.

Wagner, K.D., Ambrosini, P., Rynn, M., Wohlberg, C., Yang, R., Greenbaum, M.S., et al. (2003). Efficacy of sertraline in the treatment of children and adolescents with major depression disorder: Two randomized controlled trials. *Journal of the American Medical Association, 290,* 1033–1041.

Walkup, J. (2004). Child and adolescent psychopharmacology: What's new? Paper presented at the U.S. Psychiatric and Mental Health Congress, San Diego, November 18.

Waltman, S.H., Shearer, D., & Moore, B.A. (2018). Management of post-traumatic nightmares: A review of pharmacological and nonpharmacologic treatments since 2013. *Current Psychiatry Reports, 20*(12), 108–118

Whittington, C.J., Kendall, T., Fonagy, P., Cottrell, D., Cotgrove, A., & Boddington, E. (2004). Selective serotonin reuptake inhibitors in childhood depression: Systematic review of published versus unpublished data. *Lancet, 363*(9418), 1341–1345.

Williams, A.L., Girard, C., Jui, D., Sabina, A., & Katz, D.L. (2005). S-adenosylmethionine (SAMe) as treatment for depression: A systematic review. *Clinical Investigative Medicine, 28*(3), 132–139.

Wozniak, J., Biederman, J., Mundy, E., Mennin, D., & Faraone, S.V. (1995). A pilot family study of childhood-onset mania. *Journal of the American Academy of Child and Adolescent Psychiatry, 34,* 1577–1583.

Wozniak, J., Biederman, J., Monuteaux, M.C., Richards, J., & Faraone, S.V. (2002). Parsing the comorbidity between bipolar disorder and anxiety disorders: A familial risk analysis. *Journal of Child and Adolescent Psychopharmacology, 12*(2), 101–111.

Wray, N.R. & Gottesman, I.I. (2012). Using summary data from the Danish national registers to estimate heritabilities for schizophrenia, bipolar disorder, and major depressive disorder. *Frontiers in Genetics, 3,* 118.

**John D. Preston, PsyD, ABPP,** is a licensed psychologist, and author or coauthor of twenty books. He is professor emeritus of psychology at Alliant International University, and has also served on the faculty of the UC Davis School of Medicine. He has lectured widely in the United States and abroad. He is the recipient of the Mental Health Association's President's Award for contributions to the mental health professions, and is a fellow of the American Psychological Association.

**John H. O'Neal, MD,** is a board-certified psychiatrist who has been in private practice since 1977. He is past chief of the department of psychiatry at Sutter Community Hospital in Sacramento, CA. He is associate clinical professor of psychiatry at the UC Davis School of Medicine, and is a fellow of the American Psychiatric Association. He lectures on depression and psychopharmacology to mental health professionals, employee assistance programs, and the public. O'Neal received his master's in clinical psychology from Harvard University, and doctor of medicine from the University of Washington.

**Mary C. Talaga, RPh, PhD,** has been a pharmacist for thirty-nine years, with specialization in psychiatric pharmacy and pharmacy administration. She has extensive experience in health care, and has practiced in a variety of clinical settings. Over her career, she has contributed to the development of best practice guidelines, and has promoted collaborative care models. She has provided training and mentoring to health care professionals, and education to patients and consumers.

**Bret A. Moore, PsyD, ABPP,** is a board-certified clinical and prescribing psychologist in San Antonio, TX. Over the past twelve years, he has taught graduate-level courses in clinical psychopharmacology for multiple universities and colleges. He is the recipient of the Educator of the Year award from the American Society for the Advancement of Pharmacotherapy, and is a fellow of the American Psychological Association.

# ABOUT US

Founded by psychologist Matthew McKay and Patrick Fanning, New Harbinger has published books that promote wellness in mind, body, and spirit for more than forty-five years.

Our proven-effective self-help books and pioneering workbooks help readers of all ages and backgrounds make positive lifestyle changes, improve mental health and well-being, and achieve meaningful personal growth. In addition, our spirituality books offer profound guidance for deepening awareness and cultivating healing, self-discovery, and fulfillment.

New Harbinger is proud to be an independent and employee-owned company, publishing books that reflect its core values of integrity, innovation, commitment, sustainability, compassion, and trust. Written by leaders in the field and recommended by therapists worldwide, New Harbinger books are practical, reliable, and provide real tools for real change.

# Back Cover Material

## A Comprehensive Resource for Parents & Professionals—Now Fully Revised & Updated

*Child and Adolescent Clinical Psychopharmacology Made Simple* offers everything you need to know about the use of psychoactive medications in the treatment of childhood and adolescent psychological disorders. Whether you're a pediatrician, parent, therapist, educator, or other health care professional, this book provides clear information in easy-to-understand language.

This fully revised and updated fourth edition features new information on sleep disorders, sleep medication, and substance abuse. You'll find up-to-date information regarding teen use of antidepressants and suicidality, attention deficit/hyperactivity disorder (ADHD) and ADHD medications, bipolar disorder, psychotic episodes, and eating disorders. You'll also learn about the use of antipsychotics in children and adolescents, non-medication approaches and adjuncts to medications, and how to assess and treat noncompliance and "breakthrough" symptoms.

**For each psychological disorder, the book provides:**

- **Current DSM diagnostic criteria**
- **Treatment indications and contraindications**
- **Up-to-date medication information**
- **Help for monitoring, evaluating, and following up with patients**

**JOHN D. PRESTON, PSYD, ABPP**, is a licensed psychologist, and professor emeritus of psychology at Alliant International University. He is the recipient of the Mental Health Association's President's Award.

**JOHN H. O'NEAL, MD,** is a board-certified psychiatrist who has been in private practice since 1977. He is past chief of the department of psychiatry at Sutter Community Hospital in Sacramento, CA.

**MARY C. TALAGA, RPH, PHD,** has been a pharmacist for thirty-nine years, specializing in psychiatric pharmacy and pharmacy administration.

**BRET A. MOORE, PSYD, ABPP,** is a board-certified clinical and prescribing psychologist in San Antonio, TX. and has taught clinical psychopharmacology at the graduate level for the past twelve years.

# A

## C

www.ingramcontent.com/pod-product-compliance
Lightning Source LLC
Chambersburg PA
CBHW011302210326
41599CB00036B/7097
*9780369387103*